SPRINGHOUSE NOTES

Nursing Leadership, Management & Research

Ann Boyle Grant, RN, PhD

Dean of Instruction, Health and Science
Cuesta College
San Luis Obispo, Calif.
Adjunct Faculty
California State University, Dominguez Hills
Carson

Veta H. Massey, RN, PhD

Dean, Division of Nursing
Baptist College of Health Sciences

D1314852

Sprin

Springhouse, Pennsylvania

STAFF

Vice President
Matthew Cahill

Clinical Director
Judith Schilling McCann, RN, MSN

Editorial Director
Darlene Cooke

Art Director
John Hubbard

Managing Editor
David Moreau

Clinical Consultant
Beverly Ann Tscheschlog, RN

Editors
Karen Diamond, Peter H. Johnson, Carol Munson

Copy Editors
Brenna H. Mayer (manager), Mary T. Durkin, Stacey A. Follin, Kathryn A. Marino, Pamela Wingrod

Designers
Arlene Putterman (associate art director), Donald G. Knauss

Manufacturing
Deborah Meiris (director), Patricia K. Dorshaw (manager), Otto Mezei (book production manager)

Editorial Assistants
Beverly Lane, Marcia Mills, Liz Schaeffer

Printed in the United States of America.

NLMR-010399

A member of the Reed Elsevier plc group

Library of Congress Cataloging-in-Publication Data
Grant, Ann Boyle.
Nursing leadership, management & research / Ann Boyle Grant, Veta H. Massey.
      p.   cm. — (Springhouse notes)
   Includes bibliographical references and index.
   1. Nursing services—Administration—Outline, syllabi, etc.
2. Leadership—Outline, syllabi, etc. 3.Nursing—
Research—Outline, syllabi, etc. I. Massey, Veta H. II. Title.
III. Title: Nursing leadership, management, and research.
IV. Series.
   [DNLM: 1. Nursing—organization & administration outlines. 2. Leadership nurses' instruction. 3. Nursing Research outlines. WY 18.2 G761n 1999]
RT89.G727 1999
362.1'73'068—dc21
DNLM/DLC   98-49376
ISBN 0-87434-968-0 (alk. paper)   CIP

Contents

Appendices

Advisory Board and Reviewers

How to Use Springhouse Notes

Springhouse Notes is a multivolume study guide series developed especially for nursing students. Each volume provides essential course material in an outline format, enabling the student to review the information efficiently.

Special features appear in every chapter to make information accessible and easy to remember. **Learning objectives** encourage the student to evaluate knowledge before and after study. **Chapter overview** highlights the chapter's major concepts. Within the outlined text, key points appear in color to facilitate a quick review of critical information. Key points may include cardinal signs and symptoms, current theories, important steps in a nursing procedure, critical assessment findings, crucial nursing interventions, and successful therapies and treatments. **Points to remember** summarize each chapter's major themes. **Study questions** then offer another opportunity to review material and assess knowledge gained before moving on to new information. **Critical thinking and application exercises** conclude each chapter, challenging students to expand on knowledge gained.

Other features appear throughout the book to facilitate learning: **Insights** provide advice and suggestions on dealing with issues raised in each chapter. **Searching the Web** gives ex-amples of Web sites that provide valuable sources of additional information. **Checklists** indicate key questions to ask when evaluating leadership and management concepts or critiquing research articles.

Difficult, frequently used, or sometimes misunderstood terms are indicated by SMALL CAPITAL LETTERS in the outline and defined in the glossary, Appendix A; answers to the study questions appear in Appendix B. Finally, a Windows-based software program (see diskette on inside back cover) poses 200 multiple-choice questions in random or sequential order to assess your knowledge.

The Springhouse Notes volumes are designed as learning tools, not as primary information sources. When read conscientiously as a supplement to class attendance and textbook reading, Springhouse Notes can enhance understanding and help improve test scores and grades.

1

Overview of Nursing Leadership and Management

LEARNING OBJECTIVES

After studying this chapter, you should be able to:

♦ Describe how professional codes of ethics can provide a framework for leadership and management.

♦ Identify the steps in values clarification.

♦ Compare and contrast leadership and management.

♦ Identify the role of leadership within an organization.

♦ Identify the role of management within an organization.

♦ Discuss the historical development of organizational, leadership, and management thought.

♦ List the attributes necessary for effective leadership.

♦ Describe the functions of a nurse leader and a nurse manager.

CHAPTER OVERVIEW

Nursing leadership and management involves a complex interplay of knowledge and skills to achieve institutional, professional, and personal goals. A clear understanding of one's own beliefs and values is as essential to successful leadership and management as the ability to hire skilled staff and balance budgets, or to assist with organizational restructuring. Professional codes of ethics

1

and values clarification can help nurse leaders and managers develop an awareness of their own value systems and those espoused by the profession.

Leadership and management are related concepts, but each has specific attributes and responsibilities. Historically the development of leaders and managers has been the subject of much debate. This chapter discusses the functions and attributes of leadership and management and the relationship between the two responsibilities.

♦ I. Introduction

A. Leadership and management require a personal frame of reference; all
leadership activities and management decisions are made in reference
to a set of values and code of ethics
1. Professional codes of ethics that guide the nurse leader and manager
include the American Nurses Association (ANA) Code for Nurses
a. It provides 11 statements governing nursing conduct
b. The first of these statements recognizes a nurse's obligation to
provide services with respect for human dignity and individual
uniqueness, unrestricted by social or economic status, personal
characteristics, or the nature of the presenting health problem
2. Values clarification helps nurse leaders and managers to become
aware of personal beliefs, principles, and values so that they can examine, select, and learn to act on specific principles and beliefs
a. It helps determine the importance or significance of an experience
based on one's response to that experience
b. This process increases self-awareness and helps reaffirm a commitment to goals, increases self-confidence and autonomy, improves
decision-making skills, and guides behavioral changes
c. Values clarification can help a nurse choose a work environment
as well as personal and patient-centered goals that reflect personal
values and beliefs
d. Values clarification involves seven steps:
(1) Step 1: examining personal responses — emotional, intellectual, and physical — to experiences and interactions with
others
(2) Step 2: distinguishing between responses from internal (self)
and external (others) sources
(3) Step 3: reflecting on internal responses for consistency with
personal values
(4) Step 4: accepting the need for change in attitude or behavior
for consistency with personal values
(5) Step 5: evaluating alternative ways to achieve these changes
(6) Step 6: developing behavior patterns consistent with internal
responses and personal values
(7) Step 7: developing trust in personal feelings and intuition

B. *Leadership* and *management* are not synonymous terms
1. A leader uses specific skills to inspire the work of others
2. A manager coordinates the work of others
3. All leaders are not necessarily managers
4. Equally true, all managers are not necessarily leaders

C. An effective manager, however, is one who can identify and learn the skills of leadership

D. In some form, leadership and management are essential to all organizations

E. Understanding the nature of leadership and management within an organization requires an understanding of the organization's structure

F. An organization's structure is determined by its operative organizational theory, which serves as a basis for
1. Division and specialization of work groups
2. Number of hierarchical levels
3. Focus of decision-making authority
4. Lines of communication

G. The role of leadership within an organization is to ensure that organizational goals are attained while facilitating healthy relationships among group members through communication, group dynamics, decision making, and change

H. The role of management within an organization is to ensure that organizational goals, a reflection of organizational mission, are attained through planning, organizing, directing, and controlling

I. The roles of leader and manager are separate but can blend and overlap; they may include
1. Patient advocate
2. Decision maker
3. Educator
4. Role model
5. Change agent
6. Counselor

J. Dramatic changes in health care institutions have created a need to unite leadership and management skills
1. The nurse leader-manager must possess vision and be able to think in terms of change, renewal, and political and economic realities
2. The primary function of the nurse leader-manager is to create an environment of trust through competence
3. Nurse leaders and managers can help clarify the congruence of individual professional goals and values with those of the employing institution

4. Maintaining a position of advocacy for patients while striving for increased cost-effectiveness is one of the most important challenges in health care today

♦ II. Historical perspective

A. General information

1. Leadership and management issues have been debated for centuries
2. Elements of leadership and management can be traced through early political and governmental systems
3. The modern theories of leadership and management arose mainly from research conducted in the late 1800s and early 1900s

B. Early history to the 20th century

1. Important theorists from ancient to modern times have considered the concepts of organization, leadership, and management
2. Aristotle, in the 3rd century B.C., saw leadership as an essential component of an organized society
3. Machiavelli, in the 1500s, identified power as the basis of leadership and management
4. Adam Smith, in the 1700s, determined that effective management depends on specialization of work tasks

C. Early 1900s

1. *Classical* organizational theory was developed during this period; it holds that the role of management is to increase production by closely supervising the work of others
2. Leadership theorists of this period were mainly concerned with identifying an effective leader's traits

D. 1920s to 1960s

1. Ownership's and management's perceived lack of concern for worker satisfaction led organizational theorists to develop *humanistic* organizational theory
2. In this theory, the role of management encompasses an equal concern for production and worker satisfaction
3. Based on the work of such theorists as Peter Drucker, Abraham Maslow, Douglas McGregor, Frederick Hertzberg, and Robert House, motivating employees became a major managerial function
4. Leadership theorists of this period addressed the issues of task (work PRODUCTIVITY) and relationship (social organization of workers) behaviors and tried to predict how much emphasis should be placed on each of these issues in a given situation to achieve organizational goals

E. 1960s to present

1. By the 1960s, some theorists became concerned that humanistic organizational theory was incomplete and failed to address such issues as status and roles within organizations

INSIGHTS

Using the nursing process as a nurse manager

Nursing management, initially a daunting concept, is less intimidating when the nurse recognizes that the principles involved are very similar to those used in delivering patient care. Just as a nurse assesses a patient before setting goals, planning interventions, carrying out appropriate actions, and evaluating their results, the nurse manager assesses a situation, sets goals for personnel or groups of patients, plans the workload and organizes personnel, implements a plan of action providing encouragement to participants, and evaluates outcomes.

    2. This concern led to the development of *modern* organizational theory

    3. Modern organizational theory holds that management's primary role is to monitor communication within an organization

    4. Under this theory, leadership is viewed as a process of moving groups toward goal achievement and involves interaction among and synthesis of many variables (see *Using the nursing process as a nurse manager*)

    5. Leadership theories proposed under this theory have become the foundation for many current principles of leadership and management

◆ III. Leadership

A. General information

    1. Leadership is an interpersonal process involving influence and role modeling that inspires people to achieve personal and group goals

    2. Leadership is a learned behavior

    3. Effective leadership requires a thorough understanding of situational and group dynamics

    4. Leadership is a dynamic process that adapts to different circumstances

    5. An effective leader can assess a situation and determine the most appropriate action to attain group and organizational goals

    6. The leadership role is attained through POWER, authority, and influence

B. Attributes of an effective leader

    1. Self-confidence and self-awareness

    2. Strong personal values and the skill of values clarification, which involves choosing freely from alternatives, prizing the choice made, and acting consistently on that choice

    3. Advocacy, which involves providing information and support to those being led

    4. ACCOUNTABILITY, which involves a willingness to take responsibility for personal values and actions that affect the organization

Leadership styles

This chart lists the four most common leadership styles and representative actions and reactions.

LEADERSHIP STYLE	LEADER'S ACTIONS	SUBORDINATE'S REACTIONS
Autocratic (also called authoritative)	Exerts a strong, dogmatic direction and maintains close control over subordinate	• May feel hostile toward the supervisor and criticize decisions because staff were not included in making them
Democratic (also called collaborative, supportive, or participative)	Retains authority and control but supports subordinate's participation in setting policies and goals	• Derives satisfaction from having some decision-making control • Thinks the leader's decisions and tactics are fair because staff participated in making the decisions
Laissez-faire (also called free-rein)	Allows subordinate the chance to set goals without direction, giving subordinate maximum decision-making freedom; serves mainly as a resource	• May feel confused because of the lack of direction
Multicratic	Uses autocratic, democratic, and laissez-faire skills and styles; the choice of which depends on the nature of the situation or decision to be made	• Behaves appropriately in response to leadership when the styles chosen fit the situation; may feel leadership is inconsistent if clarity between style and situation is not provided

C. Leadership styles
   1. Leadership style refers to the behavior a leader uses in a specific situation; different situations may require different leadership styles (see *Leadership styles*)
   2. In AUTOCRATIC LEADERSHIP, the leader exerts virtually total control over group members by issuing orders, demanding obedience, and focusing on productivity
   3. *Bureaucratic leadership* is similar to autocratic leadership but places more emphasis on adhering to rigid rules and procedures
   4. In *parental leadership,* the leader fosters obedience and dependency in group members
   5. In DEMOCRATIC LEADERSHIP, the leader shares control with group members and encourages them to participate in decision making and to cooperate in carrying out decisions

6. In LAISSEZ-FAIRE LEADERSHIP, the leader relinquishes control, giving group members total freedom in a highly permissive atmosphere
7. In *multicratic leadership,* the leader moves freely among autocratic, democratic, and laissez-faire styles, depending on the situation

D. Functions of a nurse leader
1. Acts as a role model for others
2. Provides expert nursing care based on theory and research findings
3. Demonstrates knowledge about organizational theory to support and influence organizational policies
4. Collaborates with others to provide optimum health care
5. Assumes responsibility for providing information and support to patients
6. Uses advocacy to help effect changes that will benefit patients and the health care organization
7. Uses the ANA code of ethics and standards of practice as guidelines for individual and professional accountability

E. Applications to nursing
1. Health care institutions are business organizations concerned with productivity and, in many cases, profitability
2. Today, productivity in health care organizations occurs in an atmosphere of cost containment
3. Nurse leaders should focus on maintaining a high quality of patient care and on documenting and publicizing the cost-effectiveness of professional nursing in a health care organization

♦ IV. Management

A. General information
1. Management involves coordinating and supervising personnel and resources to accomplish organizational goals
2. Management functions include planning, organizing, directing, and evaluating
3. Planning, the most critical management activity, involves carefully evaluating the situation, setting goals, establishing priorities, and identifying necessary resources

B. Attributes of an effective manager
1. Sound communication, decision-making, and problem-solving skills
2. Thorough understanding of motivation, performance appraisal, quality assurance, and different management methods
3. Ability to balance sometimes conflicting goals, such as maintaining excellence in work within time and budgetary constraints
4. Vision to predict and plan for the future
5. Trust in personnel and use of group dynamic skills to achieve organizational goals
6. Concern with the task and relationship needs of personnel

SEARCHING THE WEB
Resources for nurses

NursingNet (www.nursingnet.org) provides a wide variety of resources for nurses, including links to journals, hospitals, schools, nursing unions, and specialty nursing organizations. It also maintains chat rooms.

SpringNet (www.springnet.com) offers information on resources of special interest to nursing students.

C. Functions of a nurse manager
1. Carefully assesses a situation to determine the best course of action
2. Sets goals for patients or personnel, then establishes priorities and identifies resources needed to achieve these goals
3. Structures the workload and organizes personnel to use the minimum time and resources necessary to achieve goals
4. Guides and stimulates patients or personnel to encourage adherence to the plan and progress toward goal achievement
5. Measures and documents the activity of patients or personnel as they progress toward goal achievement
6. Uses rewards and disciplinary action as components of evaluation

D. Applications to nursing
1. Health care organizations are demanding managerial expertise at the staff nurse level
2. Quality patient care hinges on effective management of a multidisciplinary team that includes professional, allied health, and unlicensed assistive personnel
3. Innovation and change, two constant factors in any health care organization, must be dealt with at the staff nurse level using communication and problem-solving to plan, direct, organize, and evaluate
4. In the ever-changing health care field, the staff nurse not only must be clinically competent but also must have managerial skills

POINTS TO REMEMBER

♦ *Leadership* and *management* are not synonymous.

♦ An effective leader possesses the qualities of self-confidence, self-awareness, values clarification, advocacy, and accountability.

♦ Different leadership styles suit different situations.

♦ Management involves planning, organizing, directing, and evaluating.

♦ The staff nurse must have clinical and managerial competency.

STUDY QUESTIONS

To evaluate your understanding of this chapter, answer the following questions in the space provided; then compare your responses with the correct answers in appendix B, pages 237 to 244.

1. What is values clarification? _____

_____

_____

2. What determines an organization's structure? _____

_____

_____

3. How does classical organizational theory view the role of management?

_____

_____

4. What type of leader fosters obedience and dependency in group members?

_____

_____

5. What is the most critical management function?_____

_____

_____

CRITICAL THINKING AND APPLICATION EXERCISES

1. Using the concept of values clarification, consider the degree to which you feel you are able to act in accordance with personal beliefs and values. Are these beliefs and values compatible with the goals of the organization for which you work? How could you constructively address areas of difference?

2. Talk with a respected nurse manager about the current emphasis on cost-containment in health care. How does the manager reconcile the professional goal of patient advocacy with the institutional goal of cost containment and profit making?

3. Appropriate leadership style may vary from one situation to another. When might an autocratic approach be appropriate? What settings might require a democratic approach?

2

Organizational Theories

LEARNING OBJECTIVES

After studying this chapter, you should be able to:

♦ Describe the three major organizational theories.

♦ Identify the theory under which most health care organizations operate.

♦ Define *bureaucratic* organizational structure.

♦ Describe the focus of a health care organization operating under a humanistic organizational theory.

CHAPTER OVERVIEW

Theories about the structure and function of organizations include classical organizational theory, developed in the late 1800s; humanistic organizational theory, which came into being during the 1920s and 1930s in part as a reaction to the mechanistic approach of classical theory; and modern organizational theory, which is based on a systems approach. Each theory describes a different vision of an organization and of the people, tasks, and environment that make up a complex organization.

♦ I. Introduction

A. The study of organizational structure is accomplished by applying organizational theories

1. The basic principles of current organizational theories have their roots in ancient times

2. Intensive research into organizational structure began during the late 19th century and continues today

B. Organizational theories fall into three basic categories, each of which is characterized by a prevailing school of thought
1. Elements of each school of thought apply to health care organizations today
2. Health care organizations are major industries and as such are structured on various principles of organizational theory

C. Organizational theories have several implications for nursing
1. Understanding organizational structures from historical and scientific perspectives provides a basis for effective nursing leadership and management
2. Nurses must be aware of the evolution of organizational theory to be able to contribute to the organization
3. Knowledge of the theory or theories under which a health care organization functions enables nurses within that organization to clarify their individual roles and functions

◆ II. Classical organizational theory

A. General information
1. The classical school of organizational theory represents the earliest attempt to study organizations scientifically
2. Many theorists have contributed to classical organizational theory
   a. Max Weber, in the late 1800s and early 1900s, developed the concept of a BUREAUCRACY as the ideal form of organization
   b. Frederick Taylor, in 1911, proposed the principles of "scientific management," which focus primarily on improving individual productivity
   c. Henri Fayol, in the 1940s, laid the foundation for the classical management functions of planning, organizing, controlling, and evaluating

B. Key concepts
1. Classical organizational theory is based on the "ideal" formal organizational structure, known as a *bureaucracy*, and on individual productivity
   a. Key elements of a bureaucracy include a centralized authority structure, highly specialized division of labor, rigid hierarchy of management, rigid rules and regulations, routine, formal communications, and detailed record keeping
   b. There is no widely accepted alternative to bureaucracy in health care organizations
2. Classical organizational theory emphasizes task orientation, efficient operation, and high individual productivity
   a. It views monetary reward as the primary incentive for encouraging high individual productivity

      b. It promotes many levels of management within an organization, with each level overseeing one specific aspect of the work and each employee developing expertise only in a particular task or set of tasks

      c. It also promotes managers' rigid, yet fair, control of employees and employees' strict obedience to those in authority

C. Applications to nursing

  1. Most health care organizations are structured based on applied principles of classical organizational theory

  2. Health care organizations have very specific chains of command, clearly delineated levels of authority, written policies and procedures, and specific rules and regulations for employees

  3. Health care organizations emphasize tasks, efficiency, and productivity in providing patient care

      a. The functional and team systems of patient care delivery are based on classical organizational theory

      b. Nurses and other personnel receive training, in the form of in-service and orientation, to develop job expertise

      c. Personnel receive monetary rewards for their work

      d. In the future, health care organizations may become more flexible structures with decentralized authority

◆ III. Humanistic organizational theory

A. General information

  1. Questions about the rigid management structure and lack of concern for employee welfare emphasized in classical theory gave rise to a new organizational theory, the humanistic (also known as the behavioral or neoclassical) theory

  2. Much of humanistic organizational theory grew out of the Hawthorne experiment, a study done between 1927 and 1933 by researchers from Harvard University

      a. The Hawthorne experiment studied certain aspects of classical organizational theory, in particular, the relationship between working conditions and worker productivity

      b. The researchers discovered that various psychological and social factors in the work situation exert more influence on productivity than do actual physical conditions; this is known as the *Hawthorne effect*

      c. The Hawthorne experiment altered the course of organizational study and moved it toward the exploration of the social climate of organizations, the "informal" organizational structures

B. Key concepts

  1. Humanistic organizational theory is concerned with formal and informal organizational structures and with the people working within the organization

2. Humanistic organizational theory focuses on group productivity, rather than on individual productivity, and on the factors that increase or decrease it

3. Central premises of humanistic organizational theory are that increased worker morale results in increased productivity; that morale and thus productivity are directly related to the social environment of the work group; and that productivity is related not only to monetary rewards but also to psychological rewards, such as group membership, a sense of belonging, and cohesion

4. Humanistic organizational theory led the way for the study of informal and formal organizational structures

C. Applications to nursing

1. The staff nurse must understand the informal and formal structures of the health care organization

2. A nurse manager's fostering of group cohesion and loyalty encourages nurses to work to capacity even when the work environment is less than ideal

3. Encouraging staff nurse participation in planning and decision making improves morale and increases productivity (see *Allow room for participation,* page 14)

4. A health care organization follows humanistic principles when it addresses employees' social needs by providing nonmonetary rewards, such as health benefits and on-site child care

5. The primary patient care delivery system (see Section II. E in chapter 4) is based on humanistic organizational theory

♦ IV. Modern organizational theory

A. General information

1. Questions about classical and humanistic organizational theories led to the development of a more modern organizational theory

2. Researchers from various disciplines have contributed to modern organizational theory

3. Development of modern organizational theory began in the 1950s with the work of systems theorist Ludwig von Bertalanffy, and it continues to evolve today

4. As a result of this continuing evolution, modern organizational theory takes many forms, including matrix theory, organic theory, technological theory, decision theory, and information-processing theory

a. *Matrix theory* stresses importance of teams built directly into the organizational structure; teams communicate and coordinate with higher management and with subordinates affected; teams have the authority to make decisions and implement them

b. *Organic theory,* similar to systems theory, stresses interrelatedness of all elements of a phenomenon; postulates that it is not possible

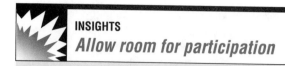

INSIGHTS
Allow room for participation

A new medical department supervisor, eager to improve cost-effectiveness and productivity, implemented a change in department structure. To allow staff to focus on patient care, she became the sole decision-maker on scheduling and ordering and the final authority on all departmental procedures. She established specific goals for each shift and provided very clear direction to staff. To avoid confusion, she established very formal lines of communication and required detailed reporting on all aspects of departmental functioning. She also negotiated an increased pay rate for all employees based on expected increases in productivity.

She was surprised when, after an initial period during which productivity did increase, staff morale declined and productivity began to suffer. Despite the increased pay rate, nurses began to request transfers to other units. When she sought advice from more experienced supervisors, she learned that professionals often function best when provided significant opportunity for input into the governance of their workplace, and that increased monetary incentives are generally not sufficient to retain staff who feel that they are unable to participate in structuring their work environment.

to deal with problems in isolation, because impact on one component ultimately impacts on the whole

c. *Technological theory* emphasizes role of technology within an organization; shapes communications and worker roles and responsibilities within an institution; provides workers with access to data more rapidly and accurately, allowing them greater control over their work and the decision-making process

d. *Decision theory* describes mechanisms an organization uses to identify problems and needs and how decisions are made based on that information; models include autocratic, democratic, laissez-faire

e. *Information-processing theory* stresses role and impact of mechanisms for assembling data and communicating information to others; describes characteristics of sender, message, and receiver, and whether information is unidirectional or bidirectional; enables examination of context in which decisions are made, and contribution of various components

5. Regardless of which form the theory takes, all can be subsumed under a *systems framework,* the hallmark of modern organizational theory

B. Key concepts

1. Modern organizational theory views organizations as complex, dynamic, social systems in which individuals, structure, end products, and environment all contribute to organizational success

a. This theory views organizations as dynamic, open structures

SEARCHING THE WEB
Nursing specialities

Information on nursing specialities can be found at Medical Matrix (www.slackinc.com/matrix). Nursing specialities have many implications for the organization of future health care environments.
SpringNet (www.springnet.com) offers information on resources of special interest to nursing students.

    b. This view of organizations differs from the classical and humanistic view of organizations as static, closed structures to be analyzed

2. Modern organizational theory focuses on organizational processes rather than on structure; these processes include INPUT, THROUGHPUT, OUTPUT, and FEEDBACK

3. This theory highlights the interrelatedness of all parts of an organization and emphasizes the need for communication and cooperation

4. The theory is concerned with the development of flexible individual roles and relationships within the organizational structure

5. Under this theory, the role of management is to monitor and coordinate communication so as to involve all parts of the system in input, throughput, output, and feedback

C. Applications to nursing

1. Few health care organizations are organized according to principles of modern organizational theory

2. When working within a systems framework, nurses are directly responsible for gathering and assessing data and planning, implementing, and evaluating all functions of input, throughput, and output; a systems approach is very similar in sequence to the nursing process

3. Nurses also must communicate to society what nurses are, what they do, why their cost is justified, and why patients need their services

4. Nurses must be comfortable with role flexibility and communication expertise to facilitate achievement of organizational goals

POINTS TO REMEMBER

♦ The classical school of organizational theory represents the earliest attempt to study organizations scientifically.

♦ Classical organizational theory is based on the bureaucratic model.

♦ Humanistic organizational theory focuses on formal and informal organizational structures.

◆ Modern organizational theory views organizations as complex, dynamic systems in which individuals, structure, end products, and environment all contribute to organizational success.

◆ Health care organizations may be structured on various principles of organizational theory; most hospitals are structured mainly on principles of classical organizational theory.

STUDY QUESTIONS

To evaluate your understanding of this chapter, answer the following questions in the space provided; then compare your responses with the correct answers in appendix B, pages 237 to 244.

1. What are three key elements of a bureaucracy? _____

   _____

   _____

2. What is meant by the Hawthorne experiment? _____

   _____

   _____

3. What is considered to be the hallmark of modern organizational theory?

   _____

   _____

4. What is the focus of modern organizational theory? _____

   _____

   _____

CRITICAL THINKING AND APPLICATION EXERCISES

1. Consider a health care institution with which you are familiar. Which of the theories of organizational structure best describes the way that it functions? How are workers within the institution viewed?

2. What advantages does an organization have when it is organized along a classical approach that emphasizes tasks, efficiency, and productivity? What advantages does a humanistic approach have?

3. How is a systems approach to organizational structure similar to the nursing process? How do nurses function within a systems framework?

3

Organizational Structures

LEARNING OBJECTIVES

After studying this chapter, you should be able to:

♦ Describe formal and informal organizational structures.

♦ Identify the four types of formal organizational structures.

♦ Describe the differences between centralized and decentralized structures.

♦ Discuss how dual structure affects nursing practice.

♦ Discuss the different types of health care organizations and the settings in which they occur.

CHAPTER OVERVIEW

The structure of an organization has a significant impact on workers at all levels. A centralized, hierarchical organization with many layers between bedside staff and decision-making administration at the top of the pyramid may provide a clear chain of command and accountability, but it sacrifices the direct communication and speed of problem solving that are possible with a decentralized structure. New forms of organization, such as matrix structures, seek to overcome these disadvantages by delegating decision making to teams built directly into the organizational structure. The expansion of corporate ownership in health care has further complicated organizational structure.

17

♦ I. Introduction

A. An ORGANIZATION is a group of people working together, under formal and informal rules of behavior, to achieve a common purpose

B. Organization also refers to the procedures, polices, and methods involved in achieving this common purpose

C. Thus, organization is a *structure* and a *process*
  1. Organizational structure refers to the lines of authority, communication, and delegation; it can be formal or informal
  2. Organizational process refers to the methods used to achieve organizational goals

D. An organization's *formal structure* is depicted in its organizational chart
  1. The organizational chart provides a blueprint depicting formal relationships, functions, and activities
  2. In the chart, the organizational structure typically is presented in pyramid form, with each level of rank subordinate to the one above it
  3. The chart designates the levels of management in an organization
  4. It depicts only the salaried employees of that organization
  5. Current trends show that organizational structure is flattening with more direct links to top management

E. An organization defines its goals and purpose in a philosophy or mission statement; this philosophy forms the basis of the formal organizational structure

F. Every organization also has an *informal structure*, characterized by unspoken, often covert, lines of communication and authority relationships not depicted in the organizational chart
  1. The informal structure develops to meet individuals' needs for friendship, a sense of belonging, and power
  2. The lines of communication in the informal structure (commonly called the "grapevine") are concerned mainly with social issues
  3. Persons with access to vital information can become powerful in the informal structure

G. Organizations also possess a unique culture of shared symbols, language, and meaning
  1. Although the organizational chart may contribute to the culture, more often, the informal, unwritten norms and values of an institution shape the culture
  2. Organizational culture encompasses both explicit and implicit expectations for standards of behavior in the workplace
  3. Organizational culture includes the sum total of the shared values and beliefs of an organization that are passed on to newcomers in the form of myths, legends, rituals, and ceremonies

H. The organizational climate, which differs from the culture, refers to how employees perceive the workplace
  1. Employee perceptions about the workplace should be consistent with the organizational culture
  2. If perceptions do not mesh with the culture, the organizational climate will be perceived as nonsupportive and unorganized
  3 Understanding the organizational culture helps the nurse expand knowledge of the norms and values of various institutions
  4. Assessment of an organization's climate helps the nurse evaluate the attractiveness of the workplace

I. The structure of a health care organization is relevant to the practice of nursing
  1. Like any organization, a health care institution has a formal and an informal organizational structure
  2. An institution's nursing department usually is structured much like the institution's overall organizational structure
  3. An institution's organizational chart depicts how the nursing department fits into the larger organizational structure and indicates the status and accountability of nurses within the organization
  4. Understanding the organizational structure helps the nurse learn the roles, relationships, and lines of communication in the institution
  5. Understanding the organizational process, including the institution's and the nursing department's philosophy, helps the nurse identify ways to achieve personal and organizational goals

♦ II. Types of formal organizational structure

A. General information
  1. Every organization creates a formal structure, which depicts lines of authority and communication and directs organizational goal attainment
  2. This formal organizational structure provides a framework for defining responsibility, authority, delegation, and accountability
  3. Depending on the organizational philosophy, the formal structure may be rigid or loose

B. Bureaucratic structure
  1. Bureaucratic structure is the predominant type of organizational structure in health care institutions
  2. This structure is characterized by many hierarchical levels and specialized positions
  3. Each level has a specific, clearly defined set of rules and regulations and scope of authority and accountability
  4. Each person at a particular level is directly responsible to an immediate supervisor

C. Functionalized structure
1. Functionalized structure is characterized by persons in specialized advisory or STAFF POSITIONS
2. These specialists enhance managerial functions by providing information and expertise to the employees of an organization but have no authority to enforce decisions

D. Ad hoc structure
1. Ad hoc structure is characterized by a more open, flexible operational mode
2. Teams are created by top-level management for a specific purpose, such as a goal or task
   a. These teams are supplementary and temporary
   b. They operate within the formal structure as a separate entity, depicted in the organizational chart as horizontally attached to the structure
   c. The teams give advice and coordinate the work of the organization

E. Matrix structure
1. Matrix structure is characterized by teams built directly into the organizational structure
   a. These teams are coordinated both vertically (within the hierarchy) and horizontally (among the groups involved)
   b. The team has formal authority to make and enforce decisions
2. Matrix structure usually involves less rigid adherence to rules and procedures

F. Applications to nursing
1. The organizational structure, as depicted in the organizational chart, provides information about status and authority relationships for the nurse
2. The placement of nursing in the organizational chart depicts nursing's status within that organization
3. Placement involves both the number and the nature of the hierarchical levels between the nursing department and the executive or top level; for example, in an organization that gives nursing a high status, the top nurse executive may be directly accountable to the chief executive officer (CEO)

♦ **III. Forms of organizational structure**

A. General information
1. An organization selects a structural form that best fits its organizational philosophy
2. Organizational structures take two basic forms: CENTRALIZED and DE-CENTRALIZED STRUCTURES

3. Depending on the structural form, the organizational chart depicts the organizational structure as a tall, pyramidal model or a flat, matrix model

4. In centralized and decentralized structures, the organizational chart delineates LINE POSITIONS, staff positions, and SPAN OF CONTROL

5. The number of management levels and the extent of span of control indicate the degree of centralization within an organization

6. Line positions refer to the formal lines of communication and authority depicted in an organizational chart by solid vertical and horizontal lines

   a. *Vertical* line positions extend from the CEO or other top official to the staff at the bottom, denoting the official chain of command

     (1) Vertical structures will diminish in height as computer information systems render them obsolete

     (2) Diversifying into new markets through the addition of services and buildings is called *vertical integration;* its purpose is to increase financial stability

     (3) Vertical management attempts to limit decentralized decision making by obtaining input from other organizational levels only on single issues of major importance

   b. *Horizontal* line positions depict the division of labor among persons with similar authority and responsibility but different functions

     (1) Merging with preexisting hospitals and health care institutions to consolidate operations is called *horizontal integration;* its purpose is to reduce operating costs

     (2) Horizontal management attempts to improve communication and decision making by obtaining input from departments that traditionally have been viewed as separate entities

7. Staff positions refer to persons employed by an organization to provide advisory assistance and expertise; these positions are depicted in the organizational chart by dotted lines

   a. Staff positions are used to enhance managerial activity

   b. Persons in staff positions have no decision-making authority

8. Span of control refers to the number of employees a manager can effectively oversee

B. Centralized structure

1. In a centralized structure, power and authority are concentrated in relatively few persons or positions (see *Centralized organization,* page 22)

2. A centralized structure has many levels or departments, each one highly specialized and subject to rigid rules and procedures

3. In a centralized structure, with its rigid rules and procedures, spans of control are short and employees and managers are in close contact

Centralized organization

This organizational chart shows a centralized nursing department and its hierarchical relationship to hospital administration. Its structure centralizes decision-making power and authority in the hands of a few people.

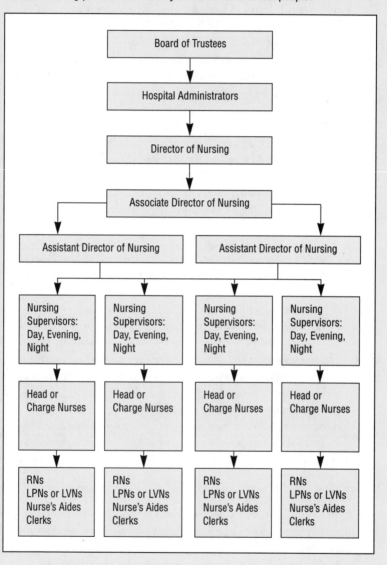

4. A centralized structure generates a tall, pyramid-shaped organizational chart depicting the multileveled hierarchy of management and individual managers' short spans of control

5. The many levels of a typical centralized structure may cause communication problems within the organization
6. In a centralized structure, leaders and managers tend to function in an autocratic management style, demanding rigid adherence to rules and procedures

C. Decentralized structure
1. In a decentralized structure, power and authority are shifted from the hands of a few persons at the top of the organizational structure to subordinate hierarchical levels
2. This structure promotes independence, responsibility, and quicker decision making at all levels of an organization
3. A decentralized structure generates a flat or matrix organizational chart, which depicts fewer management levels and wider spans of control than seen in a centralized structure
4. This wide span of control means that employees and managers have less contact with each other than in a centralized structure
5. A decentralized structure has fewer hierarchical levels than a centralized structure and tends to have better communication among levels
6. In a decentralized structure, leaders and managers tend to function democratically
   a. Managers act as resource persons rather than as authority figures
   b. Employees function more autonomously, with greater responsibility and accountability
7. Autonomy and a sense of empowerment pervade some decentralized health care institutions; as a result of their attractiveness to employees, these institutions have been labeled "magnet hospitals"
   a. Magnet hospitals embody a culture of excellence demonstrated by an atmosphere of collaboration and trust
   b. Along with decentralization, magnet hospitals use flexible models of nursing care delivery systems (see *Decentralized organization,* page 24, and *Flat organization,* page 25)

D. Applications to nursing
1. A nursing unit often is a decentralized structure operating within an overall centralized health care organization
2. A highly centralized structure usually limits the degree of autonomy and authority available to nurses
3. Bureaucratic structures remain a chief cause of job dissatisfaction among nurses
   a. To enhance nurses' job satisfaction, some health care organizations have attempted to decentralize the organizational structure by giving nurses more control over their work environment
   b. However, a shortage of nursing personnel is causing many health care organizations to return to more centralized structures, which

Decentralized organization

This organizational chart shows a decentralized nursing department and its hierarchical relationships to hospital administration. Its structure decentralizes decision-making power and authority and places it in the hands of several directors.

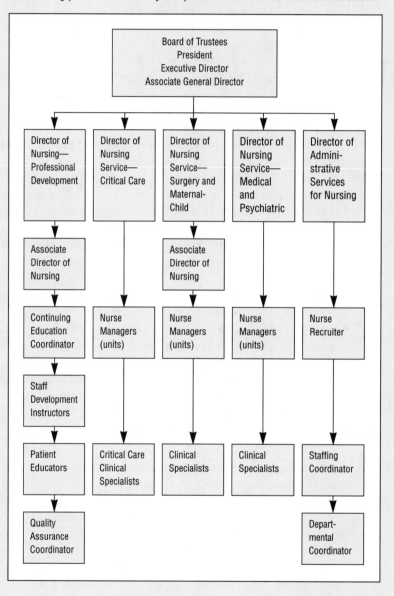

Flat organization

This organizational chart shows a reduction in the number of middle managers and a closer, more direct communication between upper-level management and caregiving staff.

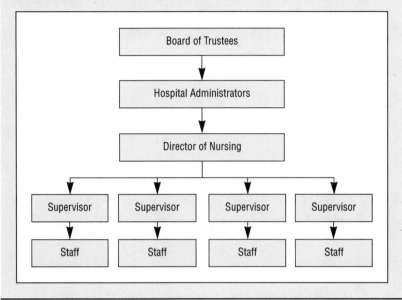

may result in greater consumer dissatisfaction with the delivery of health care services

4. Cost-containment concerns have led many health care organizations to decrease line and staff positions and to increase use of unlicensed assistive personnel

5. Health care organizations are unique in that they employ a dual structure for the medical staff, in which certain private doctors are authorized to practice within the organization but are not salaried and therefore not depicted in the organizational chart

   a. Doctors in this capacity have vertical as well as horizontal line positions; nurses are directly accountable to the organizational hierarchy but also must comply with the doctor's orders

   b. An awareness of this dual structure in most health care organizations can help nurses identify potential conflicts in authority and accountability issues and take steps to avoid them (see *Assessing the organization,* page 26)

♦ **IV. Types of health care organizations**

   A. General information

CHECKLIST
Assessing the organization

Use the following checklist in assessing the organizational structure of the institution.

	Yes	No
1. Are the levels of management clearly identified in an organizational chart?	☐	☐
2. Is there a philosophy or mission statement defining the goals and purpose of the organization?	☐	☐
3. Are there explicit and implicit expectations for standards of behavior in the workplace?	☐	☐
4. Are there lines of communication and authority within the institution?	☐	☐
5. Is there a formal organizational structure of the institution and is the position of the nursing department delineated?	☐	☐
6. Is the status and accountability of the individual within the institution defined?	☐	☐

1. The national health care delivery system includes many types of health care organizations
2. These health care organizations use various procedures, policies, and methods to achieve a common primary goal: to serve the public's health care needs
   a. This goal is achieved through administration of patient care, education of health care personnel and the public, research, and health promotion
   b. Other goals of a health care organization may vary, depending on the type and philosophy of the organization
3. Most health care organizations are formal, centralized, bureaucratic structures with definite lines of authority and communication
4. Health care organizations often are categorized by their major source of funding

B. Official health care organizations
1. Organized according to mandates from local, state, or federal government
2. Funded through governmental budgetary allocations
3. Exist at local, state, or federal levels and include city, county, and state health departments; state hospitals; the U.S. Public Health Service; and the National Institutes of Health

    4. Provide health-related and social welfare services, public works, police and fire services, agricultural services, and housing assistance

    5. Coordinate activities best accomplished through community-wide action

    6. Typically centralized bureaucratic structures but can also be functionalized, ad hoc, or matrix structures

C. Voluntary health care organizations

    1. Organized according to policies set by an elected board of trustees

    2. Not-for-profit organizations exempt from federal taxes, with operating costs covered by fees and private endowments

    3. Typically started by individuals or groups to address a specific need for service, often focusing on a single group or disease

    4. Provide health services to many people in various settings; may augment services provided by official health care organizations

    5. Usually include research and educational activities

    6. Exist at the local level (for example, a local visiting nurse association and city or county mental health associations), state level (for example, a state cancer society or state heart association), or national level (for example, the American Diabetes Association and American Red Cross)

    7. May be centralized or decentralized in form and bureaucratic, functionalized, ad hoc, or matrix in structure

D. Proprietary health care organizations

    1. Organized by their owners

    2. Provide direct health care services and contribute to health care through the establishment and enforcement of professional practice standards and funding for education and research

    3. Funded through third-party payments, fees for services, and membership fees; ineligible for federal tax exemption

    4. Include private independent providers such as medical group practices, some hospitals and institutions, and home care agencies (see *Corporate organization with multiple health care environments,* page 28)

    5. May be centralized or decentralized in form and bureaucratic, functionalized, ad hoc, or matrix in structure

E. Applications to nursing

    1. Nurses — especially nurse leaders and managers — should be aware of the structure, form, and purpose of their health care organization

    2. The nurse leader's or manager's roles and functions may differ depending on the type of health care organization in which he or she works

    3. Various degrees of autonomy and responsibility in different types of organizations make role flexibility essential for goal achievement

    4. The nurse leader or manager should apply leadership and management principles to function effectively in any type of health care organization

Corporate organization with multiple health care environments

This organizational chart shows the diversity of health care environments that may all be governed by one parent organization. Staff employed in corporate settings may work in multiple environments either by assignment or as part of a labor pool.

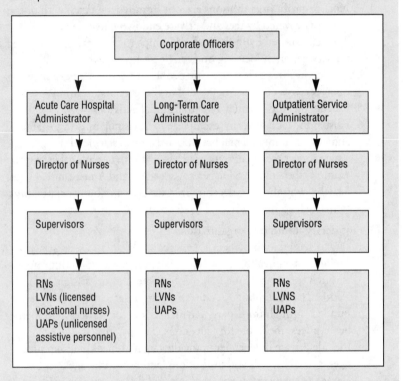

♦ **V. Health care settings**

  A. General information

    1. The three basic types of health care organizations include various health care settings

    2. Regardless of its organizational structure, form, or type, a health care organization usually is categorized by the setting in which patient care is delivered

    3. Health care organizations deliver patient care in inpatient or outpatient settings

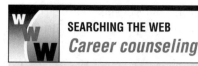

SEARCHING THE WEB
Career counseling

Nurses and nursing students can find information on jobs, resume writing, interviewing, and career counseling at the *American Journal of Nursing* Web site (www.nursingcenter.com/career).
 Springnet (www.springnet.com) offers career-related information of special interest to nursing students.

B. Inpatient settings
 1. Acute care settings, such as hospitals and trauma centers, represent the majority of inpatient health care settings
 2. Long-term care settings are growing in number as the population ages; these settings include skilled nursing facilities, nursing and convalescent homes, and rehabilitation centers

C. Outpatient settings
 1. Ambulatory care settings are either hospital-based or community-based and include surgicenters, clinics, and doctors' offices
 2. Community-care settings, including home-based care, are on the increase as a result of shorter hospital stays; visiting nurse associations and home health care agencies provide care in these settings

D. Applications to nursing
 1. Acute care settings remain the chief source of employment for nurse leaders and managers
 2. However, the increasing number of outpatient settings provides nurse leaders and managers with greater opportunities for advancement, growth, and autonomy
 3. Nurse leaders and managers need to be aware of the purpose, structure, and form of the setting in which they work to enhance the overall goals of the organization, which will ultimately lead to personal goal achievement and improved patient care
 4. A nurse leader's or manager's values and beliefs must be consistent with those of the setting in which he or she works to promote personal and job satisfaction and thereby enhance productivity

POINTS TO REMEMBER

♦ Organization is both a structure and a process. Organizational structure refers to the lines of authority, communication, and delegation; organizational process refers to the methods used to achieve organizational goals.

♦ An organization's formal structure is depicted in its organizational chart. The organizational chart provides a blueprint of the organization, depicting formal relationships, functions, and activities.

♦ Types of organizational structures include bureaucratic, functionalized, ad hoc, and matrix.

♦ Health care organizations typically are formal, centralized, bureaucratic structures.

STUDY QUESTIONS

To evaluate your understanding of this chapter, answer the following questions in the space provided; then compare your responses with the correct answers in appendix B, pages 237 to 244.

1. What forms the basis of the formal organizational structure?_____

_____

_____

2. What are the two basic forms of organizational structure? _____

_____

_____

3. What is meant by organizational climate? _____

_____

_____

4. What are three types of health care organizations categorized by their major source of funding? _____

_____

_____

CRITICAL THINKING AND APPLICATION EXERCISES

1. Obtain an organizational chart from a health care agency in your area. Does it resemble a traditional hierarchical structure? A decentralized structure? Is there more than one agency under one corporate organization? How does this affect communications and decision making?

2. Talk with a nurse manager about changes in organizational structure that have occurred over the last 5 to 10 years. What changes have occurred?

4

Organization and Delivery of Nursing Care

LEARNING OBJECTIVES

After studying this chapter, you should be able to:

♦ Identify the major components required to deliver effective nursing care.

♦ Discuss each type of patient care delivery system.

♦ Identify the types of patient care delivery systems used in centralized and decentralized organizations.

CHAPTER OVERVIEW

Patient care delivery systems have taken many forms. Case nursing, the oldest approach, involves providing care on a 1-to-1 nurse-to-patient ratio. Functional nursing, based on tasks and procedures, has been used during times of acute nursing shortages. Team nursing and primary care nursing are more recent models, which emphasize the importance of a manager or primary nurse having responsibility for patient care. Newer models include case management, in which a registered nurse (RN) or other health care professional assumes responsibility for a group of patients from admission to discharge.

♦ **I. Introduction**

   A. Delivery of nursing care is a means to achieve the goals of the health care organization

31

B. Effective delivery of nursing care promotes efficiency in an organization through high productivity and adequate STAFFING

C. Effective delivery of nursing care helps increases nurses' job satisfaction

◆ II. Types of patient care delivery systems

A. General information

1. Patient care delivery refers to the manner in which nursing care is organized and provided
2. Patient care delivery is organized at the unit level in much the same way that the nursing department and the health care organization are organized
3. The type of patient care delivery system used in a health care organization reflects the organization's philosophy; it also depends on such factors as organizational structure, nurse staffing, and patient population

B. Case nursing

1. Oldest approach to patient care
2. Involves a 1-to-1 nurse-to-patient ratio, with one nurse responsible for caring for one patient and providing all the patient care required while on duty
3. Responsible nurse reports to a head nurse, charge nurse, or nurse manager
4. Although this approach to patient care is expensive, it continues to be used in critical care units (see *Types of patient care delivery systems,* pages 34 and 35)

C. Functional nursing

1. This fragmented approach to care focuses on tasks and procedures and emphasizes efficiency, division of labor, and rigid controls
2. Functional nursing care reflects a bureaucratic, centralized organization
3. Tasks are assigned to various personnel based on complexity and required skill; for example, nursing assistants might bathe patients, practical nurses might provide certain treatments, and registered nurses would administer medications
4. Each staff member is responsible only for assigned tasks while on duty
5. The charge nurse is responsible for coordinating the activities of the unit and reports to the nurse manager; in some cases, a nurse manager may act as the charge nurse
6. Although functional nursing may be useful during times of critical staff shortages, job satisfaction may be reduced because the nurse does not see the effects of total patient care

D. Team nursing

1. Organizing patient care according to the team nursing approach reflects decentralization at the unit level and an attempt to support goal achievement through group action

2. The TEAM LEADER, rather than the nurse manager, is responsible for managing the care of a group of patients
3. Working with the team leader are various qualified personnel; these personnel report to the team leader, who then reports to the head nurse
4. The team leader assigns personnel based on their qualifications and patient needs
5. The team leader is responsible for planning and evaluating the nursing care provided by the team members
6. The nurse manager remains responsible for major management decisions, communication, and coordination for the designated unit or units

E. Primary nursing
   1. Primary nursing care reflects a decentralized organizational structure
   2. The primary nursing approach is a professional nursing model because it fosters nurses' commitment to and accountability for quality patient care
   3. A PRIMARY NURSE (an RN) is assigned to care for a group of patients throughout their hospital stays
      a. The primary nurse has 24-hour responsibility for the assigned patients
      b. The primary nurse is responsible for assessing, planning, implementing, and evaluating nursing care
      c. The primary nurse coordinates care through ongoing care plans; ASSOCIATE NURSES carry out the plan of care when the primary nurse is unavailable
   4. The nurse manager is responsible for assigning primary nurses, coordinating the activities of primary nurses on all shifts, and assigning associate nurses for periods when primary nurses are off duty

F. Contemporary nursing models
   1. In a time of economic uncertainty, health care institutions are becoming consumer driven rather than management driven
   2. The contemporary nursing approach views nurses as service providers integral to the success of the organization
   3. Newer models of workplace redesign and changing relationships between workers and management reflect this consumer-driven approach
   4. Nurses serve as case managers in many contemporary health care delivery systems; case managers may be responsible for patient care of a specific population (for example, geriatrics) or a specific specialty (for example, orthopedics) or for patients in a specific facility
   5. Independent work teams, group practice, partnership, PROFESSIONAL PRACTICE, SELF-GOVERNANCE, SHARED GOVERNANCE, stock ownership, and GAINSHARING are just a few of the new approaches that represent attempts to directly involve employees in institutional effectiveness

Types of patient care delivery systems

DELIVERY SYSTEM	DESCRIPTION	ACCOUNTABILITY FOR PATIENT CARE
Case nursing	• Based on holistic philosophy of nursing • Nurse is responsible for care and observation of specific patients • Involves a 1-to-1 nurse-patient ratio	• Nurse manager's responsibility
Functional nursing	• Based on task-oriented philosophy of nursing • Nurse performs specific tasks according to charge nurse's schedule	• Charge nurse's responsibility
Team nursing	• Based on group philosophy of nursing • Six or seven professional and nonprofessional personnel staff members work as a team, supervised by a team leader	• Team leader's responsibility
Primary nursing	• Based on comprehensive, personal philosophy of nursing • Nurse is responsible for all aspects of care — from assessing patient's condition to coordinating patient's care — for specific patients • Involves a 1-to-4 or 1-to-5 nurse-patient ratio and case-method assignments	• Primary nurse's responsibility

6. Using primary nursing as a basic structure, *case management* has emerged as a system of patient care that focuses on an entire episode of illness across all settings in which the patient receives care
   a. The nurse case manager works with case managers in other settings in a group practice structure
   b. The nurse case manager also works with doctors for each particular case type in a joint or collaborative practice structure
7. Using primary nursing, team nursing, functional nursing, or case management as a basic structure, *managed care* emphasizes achievable outcomes, effective use of resources, and cost control at the unit level
   a. Using various diagnosis-related groups as prototypes, managed care follows a time frame called a *critical path;* critical paths take into account the usual length of stay, interventions and their timing, resources needed, and expected patient outcomes

ADVANTAGES	DISADVANTAGES
• Based on comprehensive, personal philosophy of nursing • Nurse is responsible for all aspects of care — from assessing patient's condition to coordinating patient's care — for specific patients • Involves a 1-to-4 or 1-to-5 nurse-patient ratio and case-method assignments	• Increases personnel costs
• Reduces personnel costs • Supports cost controls	• Fragments nursing care • May decrease staff job satisfaction • Decreases personal contact with patient • Limits continuity of care
• Supports comprehensive care • May increase job satisfaction • Increases cost-effectiveness	• Decreases personal contact with patient • Limits continuity of care
• May increase job satisfaction • Improves continuity of care • Allows independent decision making • Supports direct nurse-patient communication • Encourages discharge planning • Improves quality of care • May increase cost-effectiveness when comparing nursing assistants' and LPNs' "down time"	• Increases personnel costs initially • Requires properly trained nurses to carry out system's principles • Restricts opportunity for evening- and night-shift nurses to participate

    b. Managed care also may rely on the use of case management plans; these plans include nursing diagnoses, patient outcomes, and the nursing and medical plans of care

8. Other responses to economic uncertainty and consumer satisfaction have resulted in various forms of differentiated practice

    a. Using primary nursing as a basic structure, ancillary personnel may be employed as nurse extenders who perform patient care tasks or clerical tasks under a professional nurse's supervision

    b. Other models of differentiated practice are based on education or assessment

       (1) In an educationally based approach, a nurse with a Bachelor of Science degree in nursing is considered the professional and nurses with less education are considered technicians

       (2) An assessment-based model differentiates staff according to ability, experience, and expertise

SEARCHING THE WEB
Resources for patients

Case managers or primary care nurses seeking information for patients and families on specific diseases can find information from several online sources. OncoLink (www.cancer.med.upenn.edu) provides information on cancer for both health professionals and lay individuals. Mental health nurses can access Internet Mental Health (www.mentalhealth.com). Medscape (www.medscape.com) provides access to the medical abstracts database of the National Library of Medicine.

G. Applications to nursing
1. Each patient care delivery system has certain advantages and disadvantages
2. The nursing shortage has caused some health care organizations to return to more centralized and bureaucratic patient care delivery systems
3. In particular, the functional approach to patient care is regaining favor because of its efficiency and comparative low cost
4. The nurse's awareness of the patient care delivery system used in various health care organizations helps guide the choice of work environment
5. To survive, health care organizations will be experimenting with new forms of organization and management; nurses must be prepared to contribute to and function in systems that reflect efficiency and quality

POINTS TO REMEMBER

♦ Effective delivery of nursing care hinges on an effective patient care delivery system and adequate staffing.

♦ Patient care delivery systems include case nursing, functional nursing, team nursing, primary nursing, and contemporary nursing models.

♦ Primary nursing reflects a decentralized organizational structure.

STUDY QUESTIONS

To evaluate your understanding of this chapter, answer the following questions in the space provided; then compare your responses with the correct answers in appendix B, pages 237 to 244.

1. Which is the oldest type of patient care delivery system? _____

_____

_____

2. Which type of patient care delivery system reflects a bureaucratic, central-ized organization? _____

_____

_____

3. In team nursing, what are the team leader's responsibilities? _____

_____

_____

4. What type of organizational structure is reflected in primary nursing? ____

_____

_____

5. What is a critical path? _____

_____

_____

CRITICAL THINKING AND APPLICATION EXERCISES

1. What would be the benefits of a functional nursing delivery system? A team nursing delivery system? Why do you think nurses have supported the move to primary care nursing and case management?

2. What is the type of delivery system used in the hospital in which you work or are training? Why do you think this particular system is in use? What advantages and disadvantages does it present?

3. Talk to members of the nursing staff at several hospitals with different pa-tient care delivery systems. How do they feel about the type of nursing practiced? Why do they feel this way?

4. What type of patient care delivery system would you feel most comfort-able working in? Why? Is this type of approach practiced in hospitals in your area? Why?

5

Theories of Leadership and Management

LEARNING OBJECTIVES

After studying this chapter, you should be able to:

♦ Discuss the theories of leadership.

♦ Compare and contrast the "great man" and trait theories.

♦ List the four elements of situational leadership theory.

♦ Describe the four styles of leadership and management in the tridimensional leadership effectiveness model.

♦ Identify the type of leadership theory likely to be found in a magnet hospital.

CHAPTER OVERVIEW

Many theories have attempted to explain the phenomenon of successful leadership. Initially, leadership was thought to be innate—some people were born leaders, and others were followers. Later, trait theory sought to explain leadership as a constellation of personality characteristics. More recently, situation theory has included environment in leadership, pointing out that successful leaders in one situation may be dysfunctional in another. Interactional theory looks at the characteristics of both leaders and followers; transformational theory examines the ability of leaders to transform workers and the workplace by building trust, confidence, and mutual commitment.

♦ I. Introduction

A. Theories of leadership and management attempt to describe and explain who a leader or manager is, what a leader or manager does, and under what conditions or through which behaviors a leader or manager can solve problems and attain goals

B. All leadership and management theories emphasize the relationship aspects and task aspects of the leader and manager roles
1. Relationship implies a concern for people
2. Task implies a concern for productivity

♦ II. "Great man" theory

A. Key concepts
1. The "GREAT MAN" theory is one of the oldest theories of leadership
2. This theory is based on the belief that a good leader has specific personal characteristics that set him or her apart from others
3. The "great man" theory posits that certain persons are "born to lead" and that leadership ability is inherited and cannot be taught or learned
4. Also according to this theory, an effective nurse leader in one situation will be an effective leader in any situation; an effective nurse leader exerts control over all aspects of a situation

B. Applications to nursing
1. According to this theory, a nurse leader attains a position based on innate leadership ability
2. A "born" nurse leader will be effective in all situations, regardless of internal or external factors

♦ III. Trait theory

A. Key concepts
1. The trait theory is based mainly on the "great man" theory, differing in the position that leadership qualities can be identified and then taught to others
2. Trait theory identifies personality traits — including intelligence, knowledge, skill, energy and enthusiasm, initiative, self-confidence, patience, persistence, and empathy — considered essential to leadership
3. The trait theory was the basis for most of the leadership research generated until the 1940s, but has been largely discredited since then
4. Over the past several decades, the shortcomings of trait theory as the sole explanation of leadership behavior and success have become apparent

5. In practice, various leadership traits have proven difficult to identify clearly and have not been useful in predicting a person's leadership abilities; studies of successful leaders have demonstrated that most had only some of the "essential" leadership traits

B. Applications to nursing
1. A nurse leader should seek to develop leadership skills and behaviors, including gaining additional knowledge through advanced nursing studies that include leadership and management topics
2. Nursing schools and health care organizations should teach nurses these skills and behaviors through didactic instruction, role modeling, case analysis, and communications review

♦ IV. Situational theory

A. Key concepts
1. SITUATIONAL THEORY expands on trait theory, holding that the essential traits for a leader vary and are determined by a particular situation
2. Based on the situation, an effective leader adopts an appropriate leadership style that emphasizes certain traits and de-emphasizes others
3. First proposed in the late 1930s, situational theory led researchers to explore the settings in which leadership occurs
4. Situational theory considers four basic elements of a situation: the *organization* (size, structure, and purpose), the *climate* (atmosphere of the organization, either supportive or nonsupportive), *leader characteristics* (power, authority, and influence), and *follower characteristics* (knowledge, dedication, and tolerance for ambiguity)
5. The leader analyzes these four elements in a given situation and chooses an appropriate leadership style
6. Appropriate leadership styles include autocratic, democratic, laissez-faire, or a combination of these styles
7. Group performance depends on the leader choosing an appropriate leadership style

B. Applications to nursing
1. An effective nurse leader will combine the best points of the three traditional leadership styles—autocratic, democratic, and laissez-faire—and, depending on the situation, use elements of all three; this approach is called a *multicratic* leadership style
2. The style used in a particular situation should be based on an analysis of the four elements of situational theory: the organization, climate, leader characteristics, and follower characteristics
3. In a crisis situation or a situation in which the followers have little or no knowledge or experience, an autocratic style of leadership may be appropriate; for example, during a code situation for a patient

with cardiac arrest, the leader takes total control, issues directives, and excludes group decision making

4. A situation requiring group input and group cooperation may call for a democratic leadership style: for example, if a nursing unit adopts a new method of documentation, the leader allows for group input to involve group members and encourage success

5. In a situation where followers are highly motivated, self-directed professionals who need little supervision, a leadership style that provides more autonomy and less direct control may be most appropriate

♦ V. Interactional theory

A. Key concepts

1. The "great man," trait, and situational leadership theories do not predict which kinds of leadership behaviors will be most effective under specific circumstances

2. A concern for measuring leadership effectiveness spawned a new approach to the study of leadership, called the INTERACTIONAL THEORY

3. Because this theory equates leadership effectiveness with high group work performance, it acts as a theory of leadership and management

4. One of the most useful interactional models for nursing is the *tridimensional leadership effectiveness and model* developed by Paul Hersey and Kenneth Blanchard, which focuses on three areas: leader behavior, group maturity, and leader effectiveness

   a. *Leader behavior* refers to various combinations of task or directing behavior versus relationship or supporting behavior

   b. *Group majority* refers to psychological and job maturity and involves commitment (defined as confidence and motivation) and competence (defined as knowledge and technical skill) to perform required tasks; the tridimensional leadership effectiveness model holds that leader behavior should be based on group maturity

   c. *Leader effectiveness* is measured by the *leader effectiveness and adaptability description (LEAD),* which includes the leader's perceptions (LEAD-self) and the group members' perceptions (LEAD-other) of the leader's style, flexibility, and overall effectiveness

5. Four leader behaviors may be used: *directing behavior,* is appropriate for a group member with low competence and high commitment; *coaching behavior,* for a group member with some competence and low commitment; *supporting behavior,* for a group member with high competence and variable commitment; and *delegating behavior,* for a group member with high competence and high commitment

6. According to the tridimensional leadership effectiveness model, leadership effectiveness hinges on choosing and implementing a

Four styles of leadership (Hersey and Blanchard model)

HIGH DIRECTIVE AND HIGH SUPPORTIVE	HIGH DIRECTIVE AND LOW SUPPORTIVE
Leader functions as coach and cheerleader, providing direction and encouragement.	Leader directs activities, providing little support
HIGH SUPPORTIVE AND LOW DIRECTIVE	**LOW SUPPORTIVE AND LOW DIRECTIVE**
Leader facilitates and encourages, but provides less direction	Leader delegates, but without direction or support

    leadership style appropriate to the task, situation, and level of group maturity

  7. Four basic leadership styles emerge from this model: *high directive and low supportive,* characterized as directing behavior in which the leader closely supervises task accomplishment; *high directive and high supportive,* characterized as coaching behavior in which the leader closely supervises task accomplishment and also supports performance through praise, listening, and facilitating; *high supportive and low directive,* characterized as supporting behavior in which the leader facilitates and encourages group members' progress toward task accomplishment; and *low supportive and low directive,* characterized as delegating behavior in which the leader allows group members to make their own decisions (*See Four styles of leadership [Hersey and Blanchard model]*)

B. Applications to nursing

  1. Interactional theory suggests that an effective nurse leader must adopt a leadership style based on accurate assessment of group maturity

  2. Leader behaviors—directing, coaching, supporting, and delegating—are required of all nurses; thus, all nurses have the potential to become effective leaders

  3. The nurse leader adopts one of four basic leadership styles—high directive and low supportive, high directive and high supportive,

SEARCHING THE WEB
Current health issues

The U.S. Department of Health and Human Services maintains a Web page (www.dhhs.gov) that provides information on current health issues from the Centers for Disease Control and Prevention, the National Institutes of Health, the Food and Drug Administration, and the Indian Health Service.

high supportive and low directive, or low supportive and low directive—at the unit and overall health care organization levels, depending on the situation, to enhance group performance

♦ VI. Transformational theory

A. Key concepts
1. In today's rapidly changing health care system, leaders are called on to positively influence both their followers and their organizations
2. According to TRANSFORMATIONAL THEORY, leaders build trust and self-esteem in themselves and others
3. A transformational leader attempts to create a workplace that is meaningful, inspiring, and motivational
4. Transformational leadership results in a workplace with a shared culture of commitment to excellence and mutual growth
5. Transformational theory is most likely to be applied in magnet hospitals

B. Applications to nursing
1. Transformational leadership is seen in health care organizations with a commitment to excellence
   a. In these organizations, nurses are rewarded for advanced and continuing education, certification status, and clinical excellence
   b. Nurses receive a yearly salary rather than an hourly wage
   c. Accountability for practice is the hallmark of these organizations
2. Decentralized organizations are crucial for the development of transformational leaders
3. Decision making and communication are shared equally in institutions that support transformational leadership

POINTS TO REMEMBER

♦ Leadership and management theories share a common emphasis on task and relationship aspects of the leader's and manager's roles.

♦ An effective leadership style is flexible and based on the task, the situation, and the level of group maturity.

♦ In a crisis situation, an autocratic leadership style may be most effective.

♦ When time allows discussion and group input, a democratic leadership style may be most effective.

♦ In a group composed of highly motivated, independent members, a modified laissez-faire leadership style may be most effective.

♦ Transformational leadership, based on trust and mutual valuing, promotes a shared culture of commitment and mutual growth for individuals and institutions.

STUDY QUESTIONS

To evaluate your understanding of this chapter, answer the following questions in the space provided; then compare your responses with the correct answers in appendix B, pages 237 to 244.

1. How does the "great man" theory attempt to explain leadership?_____

_____

_____

2. How does the trait theory attempt to explain leadership? _____

_____

_____

3. According to the situational theory, on what does group performance depend? _____

_____

_____

4. On what three areas does the tridimensional leadership effectiveness model focus? _____

_____

_____

5. What type of workplace is created by transformational leadership? _____

_____

_____

CRITICAL THINKING AND APPLICATION EXERCISES

1. What type of leadership style is appropriate in situations where time is critical and specific actions must be undertaken rapidly? Why?

2. What type of leadership style is appropriate in situations that require deliberation and cooperation of a group of educated professionals? Why?

3. Think of a recent situation in which you were responsible for the completion of a group task. How did you approach the work? What directives did you provide? What types of encouragement and support? Did you feel your approach was successful? Did your followers respond positively to your leadership?

4. Identify a case of inefficient leadership. What is the nature of the task to be done? How would you categorize the followers in terms of education, commitment, and professionalism? What style of leadership is being used? In view of Hersey and Blanchard's model, what recommendations for change would you make to this leader?

6

Concepts in Leadership and Management

LEARNING OBJECTIVES

After studying this chapter, you should be able to:

♦ Discuss the force field model of change.

♦ Describe the various phases of conflict.

♦ Differentiate between group process and group dynamics.

♦ Identify the components of upward, downward, and lateral communication.

♦ Discuss the different sources of power.

♦ Describe the role of politics in organizations.

♦ List the steps in decision making.

CHAPTER OVERVIEW

Important concepts in leadership and management include change, impetus, and direction; managing and minimizing conflict; understanding group dynamics; elements of successful communication; and the appropriate use of power and politics to advance nursing and health care goals.

♦ I. Introduction

A. The concepts used in leadership and management are derived from abstract ways of looking at certain issues

B. These concepts serve as guidelines and provide a framework for addressing the essential issues of leadership and management

C. Some concepts have resulted in models that clarify the issues

D. These concepts help apply the theories of organization, leadership, and management to nursing practice

♦ **II. Change**

A. Key concepts
1. Change is a constant in today's health care organizations
2. Various economic, demographic, and technological forces spur widespread and varied changes in health care
3. These changes may be planned or unplanned
   a. *Planned change* is an active process involving predetermined goals, participative management, a change agent, and a target for change
   b. *Unplanned change* is a reactive process whereby change either occurs without personal involvement or is introduced by outside forces
4. Planned change is initiated and guided by a skilled professional or a change agent; the change agent may be internal or external to the organization
5. The target for change may involve policies or procedures (first-order change); most change also involves the knowledge, behavior, and attitudes of others (second-order change)
6. Kurt Lewin's *force field model of change*, developed in 1951, provides a dynamic, theoretical view of the change process
   a. According to Lewin's model, in every situation two forces — DRIVING FORCES and RESTRAINING FORCES — operate in opposition
   b. Driving forces influence movement toward a goal; restraining forces obstruct goal achievement
   c. When driving forces equal restraining forces, the *status quo* is maintained
   d. Changing the status quo involves a conscious effort to increase the driving forces and decrease the restraining forces
   e. Once this occurs, planned change can take place in a three-step process of UNFREEZING, MOVING, and REFREEZING
      (1) During "unfreezing," forces emerge to threaten a planned change — resistance occurs
      (2) Next, in "moving," the planned change is implemented
      (3) Finally, "unfreezing" occurs when the new goal becomes the expected condition
      (4) Various strategies for handling resistance have been identified: POWER-COERCIVE, NORMATIVE-REEDUCATIVE, and EMPIRICAL-RATIONAL

      (a) In power-coercive strategy, power is thought to reside in the person possessing influence

      (b) In normative-reeducative strategy, change is based on the assumption that people are motivated to commit to societal norms

      (c) In empirical-rational strategy, change is based on the assumption that people are rational and will follow their self-interest

  7. The key ingredient in change is power

  8. People respond to change differently: *innovators* enjoy change, sometimes initiating changes that are not well-considered; *early adopters* tend to support and facilitate change; *early majority* respond positively, but after considerable thought; *late adopters* submit to change, but only after the majority have done so; *laggards* try to avoid change for as long as possible; *rejectors* refuse and undermine change, often in hidden ways

B. Applications to nursing

  1. Lewin's force field model of change serves as a nursing management tool

  2. Nursing leadership involves initiating changes that will enhance nursing practice

  3. Nurses also can act as change agents in efforts to restructure the overall health care delivery system

  4. Integral to this nursing role as change agent is the need for a strong power base that provides formal and informal sources of support

  5. Nurses must learn to thrive on change and become proactive, encompassing a worldview that emphasizes uncertainty and the need to cooperate with others; this new worldview is called a *paradigm shift*

  6. Strategies for creating change include communication and education, participation and involvement, facilitation and support, negotiation and agreement, co-optation and manipulation, and coercion. The type of strategy elected depends on the nature and criticality of the change, the education and receptivity of staff, and the time line for making change

♦ III. Conflict

A. Key concepts

  1. Conflict is as inevitable as change

  2. Conflict is not always negative; it can be a powerful impetus for positive change

  3. Conflict results from a disparity between real or perceived goals, values, roles, attitudes, or actions of two or more persons or groups

  4. Conflict can be competitive or disruptive

    a. Competitive conflict follows basic rules, emphasizes winning, and is usually not associated with anger and hostility

    b. Disruptive conflict does not follow basic rules and involves activities to reduce, defeat, or eliminate the opponent

5. Conflict may be *individual* (within one person), *interpersonal* (between two or more persons), *intragroup* (within a group), or *intragroup* (between two or more groups)

6. Conflict must be managed at the individual, group, and organizational levels

7. A.C. Filley's model of the conflict process (developed in 1976) explains how conflict and conflict resolution occur

8. When conflict occurs, it proceeds through various phases: perceived conflict, felt conflict, manifest conflict, conflict resolution or suppression, and conflict aftermath

    a. *Perceived* and felt *conflict* involve awareness of the conflict and feelings of tension, anxiety, and anger

    b. *Manifest conflict* consists of overt behavior, either constructive or destructive

    c. *Conflict resolution* can take one of three forms: *win-lose* in which one side dominates the other through superior power; *lose-lose,* involving resolution through avoidance, withdrawal, compromise, or bribery, with an outcome unsatisfactory to both sides; or *win-win,* involving resolution through mutual goal setting and collaboration, with an outcome satisfactory to both sides

    d. *Conflict suppression* involves repression or avoidance of conflict on direction of a higher authority

    e. In *conflict aftermath,* a person or group examines the conflict and its outcome and formulates strategies to manage future conflicts

B. Applications to nursing

1. Managing conflict is highly individualized, but skills in this area are critical for nurses

2. A nurse may be involved in simultaneous conflicts at various levels, such as with a patient, staff members, or superiors in the health care organization

3. The nurse's approach to conflict resolution creates a climate that may be constructive or destructive

4. Conflicts occasionally cannot be resolved, in which case the use of polarity dynamics may provide a way of analyzing and mitigating the effects. This involves continuing assessment of the two poles of contention, the positive and negative assessment of both extremes, and ways to move adherents of both toward a middle-road approach

♦ IV. Group dynamics

A. Key concepts

1. A *group* is an association of two or more people in an interdependent relationship with shared purposes and shared awareness

2. How a group works together to achieve goals is called the *group process*

3. The specific communication and interaction among group members is called *group dynamics*

4. Organizations consist of two types of groups: the *formal*, or work group, which has a clearly defined task designed to meet organizational goals, and the *informal*, or social group, which meets group members' needs for companionship and friendship

5. Groups tend to pass through clearly observable phases of development

   a. In *dependence* (phase I), the "forming" phase, members are insecure, anxious, and ego-centered; they feel the need for support

   b. In *independence* (phase II), the "storming" phase, members become aware of the rules and roles within the group; competition and conflict are intense; members start to view each other as a group but are still conscious of themselves

   c. In *interdependence* (phase III), the "norming" and "performing" phase, members have a strong group identity and trust and feel a sense of responsibility to and for the group; the group task is defined; rules and roles are clearly established and accepted; and group goals are perceived as more important than individual goals

   d. In *termination* (phase IV), the "adjourning" phase, the group's task has been completed and the members prepare to leave the group

6. Group size is an important factor in organizations

   a. As group size increases, so does the complexity of group dynamics

   b. An ideal work group consists of 8 to 10 members, which promotes member satisfaction and effective group process

7. All groups are guided by *group norms*—a set of overt and covert standards that shape the behavior, attitudes, and perceptions of members

8. Individual group members take on certain roles, which can be categorized as *task* (involving the job at hand and means to accomplish it), *maintenance* (involving aspects of group function), and *individual* (involving personal needs irrelevant and inconducive to group function)

9. Effective groups, both formal and informal, are characterized by strong group cohesion, in which members have a high level of attraction for one another

10. Excessive cohesion may hinder a group's receptivity to different opinions and points of view, resulting in a phenomenon known as *group think*—excessive conformity to group values

B. Applications to nursing
1. Recognizing the formal and informal work groups in the health care organization is essential for effective nursing leadership and management
2. Understanding group process and group dynamics can help a nurse become a more effective group member and group leader
3. The nurse leader is responsible for coordinating formal and informal work groups to accomplish individual and organizational goals
4. Accurate identification of a group's developmental phase can help a nurse leader confront group problems effectively
5. Confrontations should be group-centered rather than individual-centered, because a group tends to function as a whole
6. An effective nurse leader is aware of any hidden agendas—covert, private, deeply felt emotional issues that are often disruptive—that the group or individuals may have

◆ V. Communication

A. Key concepts
1. Communication involves the transmission of verbal and nonverbal messages between a sender and a receiver
   a. The sender *encodes* a message—translates it into words and gestures
   b. The receiver then *decodes* the message—translates it into a response
2. Nonverbal communication includes the components of kinesics (body motion), proxemics (use of space), paralinguistics (vocalizations such as "ah" or "um"), touch, and physical or environmental factors (heat, light, or privacy)
3. Organizations are systems of overlapping and interdependent groups structured into work, authority, status, and friendship arrangements, each with its own communication styles and rules
4. Organizational communication is a complex process that can be taught and learned
5. The many potential barriers to effective organizational communication include time pressures, environmental interference, lack of information, faulty reasoning, organizational complexity, and selective perception
6. Research has shown that 75% of all management problems result from poor communication
7. Organizational communication can be formal or informal

    a. Formal communication may be upward, downward, or lateral, as depicted in the organizational chart

      (1) *Upward communication* involves messages sent from subordinates to superiors; these messages tend to be screened at various management levels so that much of the original message is lost when it arrives at the top

      (2) *Downward communication* involves messages sent from superiors to subordinates, primarily directive in nature

      (3) *Lateral communication* involves messages sent between personnel or departments on the same level, usually dealing with task coordination

    b. Informal communication (the "grapevine") also operates through upward, downward, and lateral channels

      (1) The grapevine serves individual needs for power, personal recognition, and social interaction and may provide information not available through formal channels

      (2) The grapevine can provide rapid communication, but it also can distort information

B. Applications to nursing

1. Communication is an essential skill for the nurse manager

2. Types of communication continue to proliferate: Fax, E-mail and computers, bulletin boards, beepers and cellular phones, employee newsletters, hotlines, telemedicine communication, telephone-based triage, Internet communications

3. Nurses should attempt to overcome barriers to effective communication by establishing excellence in verbal (spoken), nonverbal (gestures and body positions), and written communication

4. Nurse leaders and managers need to practice and develop active listening skills to enhance communication

5. A nurse manager should encourage feedback from the receiver of a message to help eliminate distorted communication

6. The effective nurse manager focuses more on lateral communication than on downward communication

7. Nurses should always adhere to the formal lines of communication, as depicted in the organizational chart, to communicate within the health care organization

8. Nurses also should recognize the importance of an organization's informal lines of communication and use them to their best advantage

9. Culture has an important effect on verbal and nonverbal communication; nurses must be aware of cultural communication norms of patients and colleagues to communicate effectively (see *Beware of nonverbal communication norms*)

10. Interdisciplinary communication, such as that between nurses and doctors, is enhanced by such strategies as mutual valuing of contri-

INSIGHTS
Beware of nonverbal communication norms

When dealing with patients and coworkers from different cultural backgrounds, become aware of nonverbal communication norms, including level of speech, distance between speakers, direction of gaze, and comfort with expressing disagreement. What you may interpret as disrespect because of a soft voice and downcast eyes may actually be an expression of respect. Head-nodding, which appears to be an affirmation of understanding, may actually signal a reluctance to acknowledge, a failure to understand, or a disagreement with what has been said.

butions and collaboration in problem solving, including multidisciplinary team meetings, maintaining openness, and being appropriately assertive

♦ VI. Power

A. Key concepts

1. Leadership involves the exercise of power
2. Power, like politics, is neither inherently good nor bad despite nursing's historical reluctance to use either
3. Power is the ability to affect the attitudes or behaviors of others
4. Power is closely related to influence, which may be either direct or indirect
   a. *Direct influence* is based on role expectations associated with a given position
   b. *Indirect influence* involves role modeling, advice, guidance, and persuasion
5. *Legitimate power* derives from a formally designated position of authority
6. *Referent power* derives from the ability to inspire others' admiration of and identification with the leader
7. *Expert power* derives from the ability to inspire others based on the leader's knowledge, skill, and expertise
8. *Reward power* derives from the ability to influence behavior by granting rewards
9. *Coercive power* derives from the ability to influence behavior by withholding rewards or applying sanctions
10. Legitimate, reward, and coercive power fall into the realm of management; referent and expert power, into the realm of leadership

B. Applications to nursing

1. All nurse managers possess some degree of legitimate power—authority to carry out organizational decisions and goals

2. This authority is supplemented by the nurse manager's power to reward or coerce
3. Nurse managers become leaders through the development of referent and expert power bases that inspire others' obedience and loyalty
4. By developing referent and expert power, a nurse leader need not rely on legitimate power
5. A nurse leader can empower others by sharing power through delegation and participation in decision making; empowerment enhances self-competence and self-esteem
6. Self-competence, as manifested by clinical expertise, advanced knowledge, and expert clinical judgment, is the ultimate form of power
7. A nurse manager and nurse leader can use the various sources of power to effect change at the unit, organizational, and professional levels

♦ VII. Politics

A. Key concepts
   1. Politics refers to activities aimed at influencing others in decision making and change
   2. Politics also refers to the relationships within an organization — including procedures, values, norms, and acceptable behavior — that determine how a person will act in a given situation
   3. Politics is closely associated with power
   4. It involves using legitimate power to identify opportunities and take advantage of them
   5. Knowledge of the organizational structure, lines of communication, and individual roles and functions is essential to effective politics
   6. An organization's politics helps determine appropriate management styles within that organization
   7. Because politics is based on power, a person interested in political advancement must identify those people with decision-making power and cultivate relationships with them
   8. Because groups can exert more power than individuals, joining or organizing a special interest group can increase a person's base of power and support
   9. Joining forces with other groups who share a common interest or goal builds alliances and expands the power base to influence those with decision-making power
   10. Recognizing and rewarding those in power lays the groundwork for future assistance

B. Applications to nursing
   1. Politics in health care organizations is a means to influence people in power to promote quality patient care

CHECKLIST
Decision making

Use the following checklist to determine if the six basic steps of decision making have been utilized appropriately.

	Yes	No
1. Is the problem clearly identified?	☐	☐
2. Have all possible solutions to the problem been identified?	☐	☐
3. Have the possible consequences of each solution been analyzed?	☐	☐
4. Has the best possible solution been chosen for the problem?	☐	☐
5. Has the solution been implemented?	☐	☐
6. Have the results been evaluated?	☐	☐

2. Nurses and nurse managers can use politics to influence policy on the unit, departmental, organizational, and governmental levels
3. Staff nurses can use politics to influence policy on the unit
4. Nurse managers can use politics to influence departmental and organizational policy
5. Nurses on all levels can use politics for career advancement
6. Membership in state nurses' associations or specialty nursing organizations can help nurses participate in defining and regulating nursing
7. In this time of economic uncertainty, the allocation of scarce resources such as health care and the potential for having to ration health care takes on vast political and ethical dimensions; nurses must develop new political skills in dealing with managed care and in viewing health care as business
8. Nurses should be aware of the political and ethical ramifications of meeting not only the health care needs of individuals but also of meeting the health care needs of a society with dwindling resources

♦ VIII. Decision making

A. Key concepts
1. Decision making is a core aspect of management; every action by a leader or group springs from a decision
2. Decision making is a process of scientific problem solving that encompasses change, conflict, group dynamics, and communication
3. Decision making involves six basic steps: identifying a problem, identifying possible solutions to the problem, analyzing the possible

SEARCHING THE WEB
Health care policies and the ANA

The American Nurses Association maintains an active Web site (www. nursingworld.org) that provides information on national and state activities, policy statements, and important developments in health care policy.

consequences of each solution, choosing the best possible solution, implementing the solution, and evaluating the results (see *Decision making*, page 55)

a. Identifying problems and generating possible solutions to a problem ideally involves input from group members and tools such as brainstorming and decision models

b. Analyzing consequences and choosing the best possible solution to a problem involves such factors as cost, value, feasibility, acceptability, and risk

c. Implementing the chosen solution involves planning for contingencies to maximize acceptance of the decision

d. Evaluating the solution involves comparing the consequences of the decision with original expectations

4. Decision makers can use two basic decision-making strategies: optimizing and "satisficing"

a. An *optimizing strategy* involves examining all solutions and choosing the one that will result in the best possible outcome

b. A *"satisficing"* strategy involves choosing a solution that is not ideal but does meet minimal standards of satisfying acceptance

5. Decisions often are made under conditions of uncertainty and risk

a. *Uncertainty* implies a lack of knowledge about the consequences of a decision

b. *Risk* implies a lack of control over the consequences

6. Decision making under conditions of uncertainty is more difficult, because the decision maker has no rational basis for choosing one alternative over another

B. Applications to nursing

1. Decision making is especially important in nursing practice, when decisions often have life-and-death significance

2. The decision-making process is used by nurses and nurse managers in every facet of practice

3. Whenever possible, nurse managers should use an optimizing strategy for decision making

4. When group acceptance is important and sufficient time is available, the nurse manager should involve the group in decision making

5. The nurse manager uses the formal and informal lines of communication within the organization to gather as much information as possible to ensure optimal decision making

POINTS TO REMEMBER

◆ Change may be planned or unplanned.

◆ Conflict can be a powerful impetus for change.

◆ Group dynamics refers to communication and interaction among group members.

◆ Organizational communication channels are formal and informal and operate in upward, downward, and lateral directions.

◆ Politics and power are closely related.

◆ Decision making encompasses change, conflict, group dynamics, and communication and is at the very core of management function.

◆ Successful communications requires knowledge and appropriate use of nonverbal components.

STUDY QUESTIONS

To evaluate your understanding of this chapter, answer the following questions in the space provided; then compare your responses with the correct answers in appendix B, pages 237 to 244.

1. How does planned change differ from unplanned change? _____

_____

_____

2. What are the three potential outcomes of conflict resolution? _____

_____

_____

3. What are the five components of nonverbal communication? _____

_____

_____

4. What forms does power take? _____

_____

_____

5. What is the difference between optimizing and satisficing strategies in decision making? _____

_____

_____

CRITICAL THINKING AND APPLICATION EXERCISES

1. Shadow a nurse manager for a day, observing her communication styles, her use of decision-making skills, and her ability to use power and politics effectively. Prepare an oral presentation for classmates describing how these skills were applied by the nurse manager.

2. Talk with a patient care advocate or ombudsman. How does this individual use power to advocate for patients?

3. How do you personally feel about the use of power and politics in your role? What experiences have you had that contribute to the way you view the use of power and politics by nurses? How might you enhance your ability to use power — including political power — more effectively in your professional capacity?

7

Leadership and Management Methods

LEARNING OBJECTIVES

After studying this chapter, you should be able to:

♦ Identify the components of management by objectives.

♦ Discuss motivation as a necessary method for management.

♦ List the assumptions in a Theory X and a Theory Y philosophy of management.

♦ Identify the components of participative management.

♦ Describe the concepts of total quality management.

CHAPTER OVERVIEW

Explored in this chapter are leadership and management methods, including Blake and Mouton's managerial grid, management by objectives (MBO), and decision-making models and trees, such as the program evaluation and review technique (PERT) and the critical path method (CPM). Motivational techniques are discussed, including House's path-goal theory, McGregor's Theory X and Theory Y, and Fiedler's contingency model. Ouchi's participative management strategy (Theory Z) and total quality management (TQM) are discussed as alternatives to traditional management approaches.

♦ I. Introduction

A. Leadership and management methods refer to actions taken by a leader or manager that produce a desired outcome

B. In health care organizations, the desired outcome is quality patient care and staff productivity

C. Leadership and management methods are a means of influencing staff performance

D. The various methods serve as guidelines for motivating, encouraging, and evaluating staff with the aim of enhancing productivity, job satisfaction, and quality care

♦ II. Managerial grid

A. General information
  1. Developed by Robert Blake and Jane Mouton in 1964, the managerial grid is a widely used managerial training tool
  2. This tool presents alternative managerial methods
  3. Use of the grid helps managers evaluate their managerial styles objectively and identify areas that need improvement (see *Managerial grid*)

B. Key concepts
  1. Two key dimensions of managerial behavior are depicted on the grid: concern for production on the horizontal axis and concern for people on the vertical axis
  2. In each dimension, the manager's relative level of concern is rated on a scale of 1 to 9
  3. These two dimensions are interdependent; every manager considers both dimensions, although often to varying degrees
  4. Five basic management styles are described at the corners and in the center of the grid

C. Leadership and management styles
  1. *Impoverished management*—rated as 1, 1—is characterized by minimum concern for both production and people
  2. *Authority-obedience management*—9, 1—is characterized by great concern for production but minimum concern for people
  3. *Organization-man management*—rated as 5, 5—is characterized by moderate concern for both production and people
  4. *Country-club management*—rated as 1, 9—is characterized by minimum concern for production but great concern for people
  5. *Team management*—rated as 9, 9—is characterized by great concern for production and people
  6. Blake and Mouton proposed the team management style as the ideal

Managerial grid

The illustration below depicts a managerial grid for a nurse manager and describes the characteristics of the nurse manager for each of the leadership and management styles.

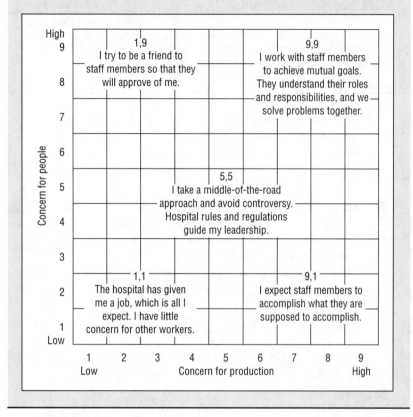

a. This style integrates and balances a concern for production and people

b. Group members feel committed to achieving group goals and individual goals; competition among group members is reduced, and communication and cooperation are enhanced

D. Applications to nursing

1. The managerial grid provides health care organizations with a means of identifying potential effective nurse managers

2. Nurse managers can use the managerial grid to assess particular situations and determine the most effective managerial style (see *Analyzing using a structured approach,* page 62)

3. Nurse managers also can use the grid to identify how their managerial styles fit particular health care organizations

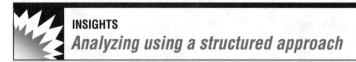

INSIGHTS
Analyzing using a structured approach

When faced with a situation where you feel your objectives as the leader or manager are not shared by your staff or colleagues, analyzing the situation using a structured approach can help you know what type of management style may work best. Understanding the type of relationship you have with the group, the degree of power or authority that you have in this particular instance, and the degree to which the task is structured can help you decide whether a task-oriented or relationship-oriented style will best accomplish your goals.

4. The team management style represents the ideal model for effective nursing management; using this approach, a nurse manager integrates concern for production and people

♦ III. Management by objectives

A. General information
1. Crucial to the management process is planning, which involves decisions about a course of action: what needs to be done, which resources are available, and who will take the necessary action
2. The management process also involves evaluation, through a mechanism of checks and balances, to ensure control over long-range and short-range plans
3. Management by objectives (MBO) is a philosophy and a method of management encompassing planning and evaluation
4. Introduced by Peter Drucker in 1954, MBO was designed to improve employee morale and productivity

B. Key concepts
1. MBO provides a mechanism for establishing measurable goals throughout an organization
2. MBO emphasizes self-control rather than managerial control of employee behavior and stresses teamwork
3. Employees establish individual standards of performance and expected outcomes based on organizational goals
4. Goals are formulated at all levels: organizational, departmental, unit, and individual
5. MBO is a three-step process: writing clear, concise, measurable objectives; developing a plan to meet the objectives; and evaluating the plan at predetermined times and taking corrective action if necessary
6. MBO results in better organizational planning

C. Leadership and management styles

1. In MBO, management facilitates employee development and achievement
2. The manager focuses on employees' measurable objectives rather than on their personal characteristics
3. The manager is responsible for employee development through setting standards of quality performance, providing well-timed feedback, and giving sufficient rewards
4. MBO is used less frequently by managers who subscribe to a TOTAL QUALITY MANAGEMENT philosophy (see Section X, page 71)

D. Applications to nursing

1. Most health care organizations operate under some form of MBO because it provides an effective and consistent method of performance evaluation
2. Nurses should be aware of their organizational mission, purpose, and goals and their departmental and unit goals when developing their own objectives
3. MBO places great emphasis on the attributes of values clarification and accountability
4. In determining plans and aspirations, the nurse manager develops a written list of objectives and priorities and time frames for accomplishing objectives
5. In this list, objectives should be realistically stated and should encourage personal and professional growth by promoting increased self-awareness, accountability, satisfaction, and productivity

◆ IV. Decision-making models and trees

A. General information

1. Decision-making models and trees can generate solutions to a problem
2. Decision-making models use DECISION TREES to solve problems
3. Decision trees diagram the problem-solving process

B. Key concepts

1. A decision tree depicts a problem, alternative solutions to the problem, and possible consequences of each solution ranked by the risk or probability of occurrence
2. The problem must have at least two solutions
3. As solutions are listed, the decision-making process "branches out" to resemble a tree
4. Decision-making models include program evaluation and review technique, critical path method, and normative decision making
   a. The *program evaluation and review technique* (PERT) is a network system model of decision making, problem solving, and planning that determines priorities through key activities, time progression,

and flow of events; it is frequently used in construction projects in health care or in major reorganizations

b. The *Critical path method* (CPM), an aspect of PERT, diagrams the order in which tasks are to be accomplished or completed; this process should not be confused with clinical pathways, which deal with patient progress and outcomes

c. The *Vroom and Yetton normative decision-making model,* developed in 1973, examines specific managerial decision styles

(1) It examines seven problem attributes: the importance of the quality of the decision, the manager's knowledge or expertise, the group's knowledge or expertise, the problem structure, the importance of the group's acceptance of the decision, the group's acceptance of an autocratic decision, and the group's commitment to organizational goals

(2) Decision styles are determined by how the seven DECISION RULES apply to a specific situation

(3) The seven decision rules are the information rule, the goal congruence rule, the unstructured problem rule, the acceptance rule, the conflict rule, the fairness rule, and the acceptance priority rule

C. Leadership and management styles

1. Vroom and Yetton identified five main managerial decision styles: autocratic I, autocratic II, consultative I, consultative II, and group II

2. *Autocratic I decision style:* the manager solves the problem or makes the decision using information available only to himself or herself

3. *Autocratic II decision style:* the manager lacks the information necessary to solve the problem and obtains it from subordinates; the subordinates provide information only about the problem and do not generate or evaluate alternative solutions

4. *Consultatitve I decision style:* the manager shares the problem with subordinates individually, then makes a decision that may or may not reflect their input

5 *Consultative II decision style:* the manager shares the problem with subordinates as a group, then makes a decision that may or may not reflect group input

6. *Group II decision style:* the manager shares the problem with the group, and together they propose solutions; the manager does not try to influence the group and is willing to implement any solution supported by the group even if it is not the manager's chosen solution (see *Decision rules and decision styles*)

D. Applications to nursing

1. Decision-making models and trees provide the nurse manager with a quick and effective means of decision making

Decision rules and decision styles

This chart lists the seven decision rules of the Vroom and Yetton decision-making model and describes them in terms of problem attributes. It then identifies possible decision styles based on the decision rules and problem attributes.

DECISION RULE	PROBLEM ATTRIBUTES CONSIDERED	POSSIBLE DECISION STYLES
Information rule	• Quality of decision is important • Manager lacks information to solve the problem	Autocratic II, Consultative I, Consultative II, Group II
Goal congruence rule	• Quality of decision is important • Subordinates lack shared commitment to organizational goals	Autocratic I, Autocratic II, Consultative I, Consultative II
Unstructured problem rule	• Quality of decision is important • Leader lacks information to solve problem • Problem lacks structure • Interaction among subordinates is important	Consultative II, Group II
Acceptance rule	• Subordinate acceptance is important • Autocratic decision is unacceptable • Subordinate participation is important	Consultative I, Consultative II, Group II
Conflict rule	• Subordinate acceptance is important • Autocratic decision is unacceptable • Subordinates are likely to disagree over decision	Consultative II, Group II
Fairness rule	• Quality of decision is unimportant • Subordinate acceptance is important to implement decision • Autocratic decision is unacceptable	Group II
Acceptance priority rule	• Subordinate acceptance is important to implement decision • Autocratic decision may not be acceptable • Subordinates are allowed to participate in decision making	Group II

2. A nurse manager can use this method of problem solving at the unit and organizational levels
3. A nurse manager should carefully assess a problem and consult with staff members to determine the most effective solution

4. A nurse manager must examine an alternative solution's possible consequences and risks carefully to ensure that the decision minimizes loss and maximizes gain
5. A nurse manager who is aware of organizational and unit objectives can solve problems effectively

♦ V. Motivation

A. General information
1. To achieve established goals, persons must be motivated
2. Motivated behavior is goal-directed behavior
3. Motivating employees to achieve goals is a crucial managerial skill
4. The Hawthorne experiment (see Section III. A in Chapter 2) ushered in a new era of management that focused on concern for production and employees
5. Subsequent research into MOTIVATION resulted in motivational theories; major motivational theorists include Abraham Maslow, David McClelland, and Frederick Herzberg

B. Key concepts
1. All motivational theories have common threads: concern for what causes human behavior, what directs behavior toward goal accomplishment, and what encourages this behavior over time
2. Maslow described motivation as the innate impetus to satisfy what he termed the hierarchy of human needs: biological needs, safety needs, need for love and sense of belonging, need for self-esteem, and need for self-actualization
3. McClelland, elaborating on Maslow's hierarchy, identified three motivational needs present in varying degrees in all persons operating in an organizational setting: achievement, affiliation, and control
4. Herzberg's two-factor theory discusses motivation in terms of job satisfaction
   a. The lack of such external factors as adequate salary, job security, and decent working conditions leads to job dissatisfaction and poor work performance
   b. Job satisfaction results mainly from promoting internal factors such as recognition, respect, authority, and status

C. Leadership and management styles
1. The effective motivational manager diagnoses human needs
2. The manager must also diagnose situations, because human needs (and thus the optimal motivational strategy) vary in different situations
3. Motivating employees depends not only on satisfying needs for a safe and secure environment but also on satisfying needs for self-esteem, self-actualization, and achievement

4. The manager recognizes competent work by providing objective feedback and recognition for performance, which motivate continued productivity

D. Applications to nursing
1. Health care organizations use motivation to achieve organizational goals
2. Nurse managers use motivation in daily practice
3. Nurse managers use motivational strategies when leading a team or caring for a group of patients
4. To motivate people, nurse managers must identify their own needs and expectations
5. Nurse managers should set reasonable work goals and reward staff for work well done
   a. A motivated work group has a clear definition of tasks and promotes a friendly, supportive atmosphere
   b. Staff must be challenged to develop expertise and pride in their work

♦ **VI. Path-goal theory**

A. General information
1. Robert House's path-goal theory, introduced in 1971, is concerned with motivation and productivity
2. It attempts to evaluate the effect of the leader on group members
3. According to this theory, the motivational function of management is to help employees see the relationship between personal and organizational goals, clarify the "paths" to accomplishing these goals, remove obstacles to goal achievement, and reward employees for work accomplished

B. Key concepts
1. According to this theory, an effective leader or manager clarifies the path to the goal by structuring the work through planning, organizing, directing, and controlling
2. Structuring the work increases employee productivity
3. The manager who shows considerate behavior toward employees, engaging in supportive, warm, and friendly relationships with them, helps promote employees' job satisfaction

C. Leadership and management styles
1. An effective leader or manager adopts a specific behavioral style to increase employee motivation and productivity
2. *Supportive behavior* considers the needs of employees and fosters a friendly work environment
3. *Directive behavior* clarifies the path to the goal by structuring the necessary tasks

4. *Achievement-oriented behavior* challenges employees to strive for excellence

5. *Participative behavior* engages employees in decision making

D. Applications to nursing

1. A nurse manager's supportive behavior is especially important for employees engaged in routine nursing tasks

2. A nurse manager can use directive behavior to demonstrate the relationship between performance and reward and thus improve employee motivation

3. A nurse manager can use achievement-oriented behavior to challenge staff members to attain excellence in job performance

4. A nurse manager can use participative behavior to obtain staff input and cooperation in making decisions about goals and how they are to be accomplished

5. The use of outcome management, which focuses on processes and outcomes rather than tasks, helps build effective, collaborative work behaviors

♦ VII. Theory X and Theory Y

A. General information

1. The directing and evaluating functions of management are shaped by managers' assumptions about their employees

2. Douglas McGregor, in 1960, labeled these assumptions Theory X and Theory Y

3. Depending on which set of assumptions the manager subscribes to, the amount of direction and control given to employees will vary

B. Key concepts

1. *Theory X* assumes that people dislike work and must be directed, controlled, and coerced into working productively; that people will resist authority and responsibility; and that they work only for security and economic rewards

2. A Theory X–oriented manager emphasizes organizational goals

3. *Theory Y* assumes that people are creative and imaginative and will achieve satisfaction from work and that people are self-directed and self-controlled and will accept responsibility under favorable conditions

4. A Theory Y–oriented manager emphasizes individual goals

5. McGregor believed that each approach is ineffective by itself and, as such, recommended a restructuring of the workplace so that true collaboration can occur while meeting individual goals and working toward organizational goals

C. Leadership and management styles

1. According to Theory X, a manager should be autocratic, directive, and task-oriented and solicit little input from subordinates

2. According to Theory Y, a manager should be democratic, supportive, and relationship-oriented and should delegate to and accept input from subordinates

D. Applications to nursing
1. A nurse manager with a Theory X orientation will allow for minimal
employee input, delegate little, supervise closely, and comply strictly
with rules and regulations
2. A nurse manager with a Theory Y orientation will encourage employee input, provide loose supervision, delegate responsibilities,
and allow for personal expression

♦ VIII. Contingency model

A. General information
1. Introduced by Fred Fiedler in 1967, the contingency model of managerial effectiveness is based on group productivity
2. Although this is a management model, it uses the terms *leader* and
leadership
3. The leader has primary responsibility for the group and has the
power and influence to ensure that the group works effectively
4. Defining leadership as a relationship involving power and influence,
Fiedler explored how much power and influence situations provide
the leader
5. The contingency model highlights the need for flexibility in leadership behaviors
6. The validity of the contingency model has been supported by effective research

B. Key concepts
1. In the contingency model, three situational variables are used to predict the favorability of a situation for the leader: the leader's interpersonal relations with group members, the leader's LEGITIMATE POW-
ER, and the task structure
2. These three variables produce eight situations ranked from "most favorable" to "least favorable" in terms of their effect on the leader;
each of these eight situations is numbered and referred to as a cell
3. Cells 1, 2, 3, and 8 are the most favorable and least favorable situations for the leader, calling for a controlling, autocratic leadership
style; cells 4 and 5 are moderately favorable situations, calling for a
permissive, democratic leadership style; and cells 6 and 7 are unfavorable situations calling for either a permissive or controlling leadership style

C. Leadership and management styles
1. When relationships with the group are good, the work is structured,
and the leader is powerful (cell 1), a task-oriented style is best

2. When relationships with the group are good, the work is structured, and the leader has weak power (cell 2), a task-oriented style is best
3. When relationships with the group are good, the work is unstructured, and the leader is powerful (cell 3), a task-oriented style is best
4. When relationships with the group are poor, the work is unstructured, and the leader has weak power (cell 8), a task-oriented style is best
5. When relationships with the group are good, the work is unstructured, and the leader has weak power (cell 4), a relationship-oriented style is best
6. When relationships with the group are poor, the work is structured, and the leader is powerful (cell 5), a relationship-oriented style is best
7. When relationships with the group are poor, the work is structured, and the leader has weak power (cell 6), a relationship-oriented style is best
8. When relationships with the group are poor, the work is unstructured, and the leader is powerful (cell 7), a relationship-oriented style is best

D. Applications to nursing
1. According to the contingency model, a nurse manager should modify situations based on group relations, personal power, and task structure to improve staff productivity
2. A nurse manager who uses the contingency model must have a thorough understanding of his or her relationship with staff members, his or her power and status within the organization, and the nature of the group task
3. Based on this assessment, the nurse manager can describe the situation as favorable, moderately favorable, or unfavorable
   a. In favorable and unfavorable situations, the nurse manager should adopt a task-oriented approach
   b. In moderately favorable situations, a relationship-oriented approach is best

♦ IX. Participative approach to management (Theory Z)

A. General information
1. Participative management involves a collaborative approach
2. William Ouchi's Theory Z, introduced in 1981, is one form of participative management that focuses on ways to motivate workers and thereby increase employee job satisfaction and improve productivity
3. Participative management combines the elements of MBO, motivational principles, and employee enhancement

4. Participative management is based on identification of organizational structure and policies, employees' needs and motivations, and measurements of productivity

5. Participative management integrates the formal and informal structures of the organization through shared goal setting

B. Key concepts

1. Overall organizational goals are set by top management

2. Groups involved in participative management have an appointed leader

3. The leader is granted authority for problems falling under his or her jurisdiction

4. Participative management is characterized by "quality circles," which involve group decision making

5. In participative management, decentralized organizational structure, MBO, and group decision making effectively transfer power to the level at which individual decisions must be made

6. Working under a system of participative management requires shared authority, responsibility, and accountability

7. The success of participative management hinges on managers' and employees' commitment to the organization

C. Leadership and management styles

1. Participative management requires that managers have good leadership qualities, because it integrates leadership and management

2. It promotes a relationship-oriented, democratic leadership style

3. The leader supports employee achievement and relies on delegating and supporting leadership styles

D. Applications to nursing

1. Participative management provides a professional model for nursing care

2. Primary nursing is an essential component of participative management

3. Participative management supports decision making at the unit level, thereby fostering accountability

4. Implementing participative management requires thorough staff education and frequent feedback on progress

5. Nurses involved in this type of management model are responsible for implementing goals at the unit level; they should be committed to nursing as a career

♦ X. Total quality management

A. General information

1. Total quality management (TQM) is a philosophy of management developed by W. Edwards Deming

2. Originally implemented in Japan after World War II, TQM is credited with the outstanding recovery of postwar Japanese industry
3. TQM was introduced to various organizations in the United States in the 1970s
4. Almost 70% of those organizations failed in their attempts to implement TQM
5. Continuous quality improvement (CQI) is a recent outgrowth of TQM

B. Key concepts
1. Employees are given more authority over their work in a TQM system; individual employees have autonomy in decision making (for a TQM checklist, see *Total quality management method*)
2. Employees are trained to make decisions that improve both the quality of the work and the productivity of the workers
3. TQM embodies a paradigm shift from an emphasis on monitoring quality through scientific data collection to an ongoing, continuous measuring of quality through human responses to care
4. Strategic planning for the future through the establishment of a long-term commitment to productivity and quality is the key to TQM
5. TQM attempts to address the need for productivity and quality by meeting the concerns of both internal (employees) and external (patients) customers; organizational teamwork and individual empowerment are essential
6. The focus of TQM is on results rather than on daily activities and on improving processes rather than identifying fault
7. Ongoing evaluation of progress is an essential component of TQM

C. Application to nursing
1. The philosophy of TQM is summarized in Deming's "14 points" (see *Fourteen points to the Deming management method,* page 74)
2. Some hospitals are attempting to translate TQM into a model for management and the Joint Commission on Accreditation of Healthcare Organizations (JCAHO) stresses the use of processes such as CQI
3. A shared governance structure within the nursing department best supports the management processes outlined by TQM
4. TQM requires major system changes, including adoption of new organizational values
5. It takes at least 5 years to adopt an organizational culture that promotes individual accountability and excellence
6. The primary reason that so many industries, including health care organizations, fail to successfully implement TQM is management's reluctance to relinquish power and control

CHECKLIST
Total quality management method

Use the following questions to critique the commitment of the institution to productivity and quality enhancement methods within the management framework.

	Yes	No
1. Is there a statement of the aims and purposes of the company published to all employees and does management consistently demonstrate their commitment to this statement?	☐	☐
2. Is the philosophy of the company known by everyone (top management and every employee) alike?	☐	☐
3. Are inspections performed for the purpose of improvement of processes and reduction of costs?	☐	☐
4. Is business awarded on a basis other than price tag? Is the system of production and service constantly being improved upon?	☐	☐
5. Is training instituted?	☐	☐
6. Is leadership taught and instituted?	☐	☐
7. Is a climate for trust created as well as a climate for innovation?	☐	☐
8. Are the efforts of teams, groups, and staff areas optimized toward the aims and purposes of the company?	☐	☐
9. Are exhortations for the work force eliminated?	☐	☐
10. Are numerical quotas for production eliminated and replaced with instituted methods for improvement?	☐	☐
11. Is Management by Objective eliminated and replaced with improving upon the capabilities of processes?	☐	☐
12. Are barriers removed that rob people of pride and workmanship?	☐	☐
13. Is education and self improvement encouraged for everyone?	☐	☐
14. Is action taken to accomplish the transformation?	☐	☐

7. Effective use of TQM requires education of nurses in school curricula or institutional settings, particularly with regard to the nurse's role on TQM teams

8. Effective use of TQM requires adequate budgetary support as well as staffing support for nurses to serve on TQM teams

Fourteen points to the Deming management method

1. Create and publish to all employees a statement of the aims and purposes of the company or other organization. The management must demonstrate constantly their commitment to this statement.
2. Learn the new philosophy, top management and everybody.
3. Understand the purpose of inspection, for improvement of processes and reduction of cost.
4. End the practice of awarding business on the basis of price tag alone.
5. Improve constantly and forever the system of production and service.
6. Institute training.
7. Teach and institute leadership.
8. Drive out fear. Create trust. Create a climate for innovation.
9. Optimize toward the aims and purposes of the company the efforts of teams, groups, staff areas.
10. Eliminate exhortations for the work force.
11a. Eliminate numerical quotas for production. Instead, learn and institute methods for improvement.
11b. Eliminate management by objective. Instead, learn the capabilities of processes and how to improve them.
12. Remove barriers that rob people of pride of workmanship.
13. Encourage education and self-improvement for everybody.
14. Take action to accomplish the transformation.

Reprinted from *Out of the Crisis* by W. Edwards Deming with permission from MIT and The W. Edwards Deming Institute. Published by MIT, Center for Advanced Educational Services, Cambridge, MA 02139. Copyright 1986 by The W. Edwards Deming Institute.

POINTS TO REMEMBER

◆ Management by objectives is both a management philosophy and a management method.

◆ Decision-making models and trees provide effective approaches to problems.

◆ Motivating employees is an important managerial skill.

◆ Motivation derives from such factors as status, recognition, self-actualization, and affiliation.

◆ According to the path-goal theory, the motivational function of management is to help employees see the relationship between personal and organizational goals, clarify the paths to accomplishing these goals, remove obstacles to goal achievement, and reward employees for work accomplished.

- The directing and evaluating functions of management are shaped by managers' assumptions about their employees — assumptions that Douglas McGregor labeled Theory X and Theory Y.

- The contingency model highlights the need for flexibility in leadership and management style.

- Participative management decentralizes authority to the unit level.

- Total quality management monitors quality through human responses to care.

STUDY QUESTIONS

To evaluate your understanding of this chapter, answer the following questions in the space provided; then compare your responses with the correct answers in appendix B, pages 237 to 244.

1. According to the managerial grid, which management style is considered the most effective and why? _____

_____

_____

2. How are various management styles related to employee motivation?

_____

_____

3. Which model of management uses the concept of power in predicting the favorability of various situations for the manager? _____

_____

_____

4. Which type of overall organizational structure is crucial to a participative approach to management? _____

_____

_____

5. What factors are essential to successful implementation of a total quality management approach? _____

_____

_____

CRITICAL THINKING AND APPLICATION EXERCISES

1. Identify a project requiring the support of coworkers. How could you build motivation in these individuals? What supportive behaviors could you use? Directive behaviors? Achievement-oriented behaviors? Participative behaviors?

2. Identify a nurse who you feel exemplifies an effective leader. How would you analyze the leadership and management style as defined by Blake and Mouton? Using the description of styles and characteristics on page 60, place this leader on the grid. Why do these characteristics make this nurse a successful leader and manager?

3. Examine your own leadership and management. Where do you fit on the grid on page 61? Are you more concerned with people or production? What does this imply for your working relationships? Your ability to accomplish goals?

8

Processes in Leadership and Management

LEARNING OBJECTIVES

After studying this chapter, you should be able to:

♦ Identify the characteristics of an assertive person.

♦ Discuss the components of time management and common barriers to utilization.

♦ Describe the elements of performance appraisal and quality assurance.

♦ Identify the four components of an effective marketing plan.

♦ Define *networking*.

♦ Describe the process of mentoring.

♦ Discuss the nurse manager's role in risk management.

♦ Identify the important components of team building, leading meetings, and interviewing.

CHAPTER OVERVIEW

Effective leadership and management include such important skills and processes as assertiveness, time management, and performance appraisal. Ongoing assessment of work processes and outcomes is accomplished through

77

quality assurance and continuous quality improvement (CQI). Successful managers and leaders also use marketing, networking, mentoring, and risk management processes. Other important skills include stress management, team building, and interviewing.

♦ I. Introduction

A. Processes used in leadership and management refer to those actions that enable a person to become a leader or manager or to improve skills

B. These processes incorporate important leadership and management concepts and methods

♦ II. Assertiveness

A. Key concepts
1. Assertiveness is a process of communicating with self-confidence
2. It involves a balance between passiveness and aggressiveness
3. Assertiveness can be learned
4. An assertive person stands up for his or her rights but is careful not to infringe on the rights of others
5. An assertive person expresses feelings and needs clearly, honestly, and respectfully through I-MESSAGES, so that others have no doubts as to how their behavior affects the assertive person
6. An assertive person faces problems squarely and suggests solutions

B. Applications to nursing
1. A nurse leader or manager must be assertive to facilitate problem identification, problem solving, and decision making
2. A nurse leader or manager uses assertiveness to communicate staff needs to superiors
3. Assertive behavior by a nurse leader or manager often encourages staff to respond in the same fashion, promoting goal achievement
4. On a personal level, a nurse leader or manager can use assertiveness to manage stress, achieve a positive self-image, and improve professional productivity and job satisfaction
5. Appropriate assertive behaviors are essential in effective advocacy for patients
6. Appropriate assertive behaviors assist in channeling anger toward solutions

♦ III. Time management

A. Key concepts
1. Time management involves planning and scheduling for anticipated and unanticipated events in the workday
2. Effective time management hinges on priority setting and delegation

a. Priority setting involves classifying activities and determining the optimal order in which they should be performed

b. Delegation involves assigning duties and responsibilities to properly prepared subordinates and making these subordinates accountable for their performance; unlicensed assistive personnel (UAPs) require proper training, certification, supervision, and evaluation

3. Barriers to effective time management include interruptions and distractions, such as phone calls and visitors; learning to manage these interruptions is vital for effective time management

B. Applications to nursing

1. Time management skills must be learned; nurses should seek out opportunities in work and educational settings to develop these skills, which are necessary for working efficiently and providing optimal patient care

2. Priorities for organizational goals are identified by a nurse manager's superiors and then delegated to the nurse manager for completion

3. Priorities for personal and unit goals are identified by a nurse manager

4. A nurse manager delegates duties and responsibilities to staff nurses, who in turn delegate duties and responsibilities to ancillary staff

5. A nurse manager who delegates to a staff nurse must give the staff nurse authority to perform the task

6. When a nurse manager delegates effectively, both the nurse manager and the subordinate are accountable for the result

7. Effective use of time management skills requires provision of necessary tools, equipment, and environmental supports

8. Formal meetings and discussions should be set up by the nurse manager with a clear purpose, agenda, and time limit in mind, to minimize or prevent interruptions and distractions

♦ IV. Performance appraisal

A. Key concepts

1. Performance appraisal is an integral part of management and provides an effective method of motivating employees and improving work performance

2. It involves periodic evaluation of the strengths and weaknesses of a worker's job performance and is conducted by the worker's supervisor (who typically holds a line position in the organization)

3. It involves objective and subjective factors

a. *Objective factors* are measurable behaviors, such as lateness and absences

b. *Subjective* factors are behaviors related to job performance, which the evaluator appraises and rates, usually using a checklist or rating scale; emphasis should be on observable behaviors and not on personality factors

B. Applications to nursing

  1. Nurse managers need in-depth training in performance appraisal to avoid bias and prejudice

  2. Assessment of a staff nurse's performance should be ongoing; this should be a formal process, utilizing a set appointment time and thereby avoiding surprises

  3. Corrective action, if necessary, should focus on helping the staff nurse set goals for improved performance; progressive discipline, if improvement does not occur, involves a step-by-step method of addressing ongoing problems

  4. The nurse manager can select the best example of a nurse's performance and apply that example as a standard to improve performance; this is known as *benchmarking*

  5. Performance appraisal should involve identification of positive as well as negative elements and should be done supportively with staff nurse participation

♦ V. Quality assurance

A. Key concepts

  1. In health care, quality assurance is an evaluation of patient care

  2. Quality assurance includes self-evaluation, performance appraisal, peer review, audits, and utilization review; it provides accountability at the individual, unit, and organizational levels

  3. The need for quality assurance in health care has intensified with rising costs

  4. In hospitals, quality assurance programs are based on outcome and process standards established by the American Nurses Association (ANA), the American Hospital Association, and the Joint Commission on Accreditation of Health Care Organizations (JCAHO); the Occupational Safety and Health Administration provides standards for the establishment and enforcement of health and safety protocols to protect employees in the workplace.

  5. Quality assurance initially focused on the cost and quality of care received by patients in the Medicare, Medicaid, and maternal-child health programs

  6. Quality assurance programs focus on *structure*, the setting in which patient care is delivered; *process*, the manner in which care is delivered; and *outcome*, the results of that care

  7. Quality assurance involves setting STANDARDS, establishing criteria, and evaluating performance

    a. Setting standards involves the ANA Standards of Nursing Practice and specific standards or objectives for the patient population

       b. Establishing criteria involves determining how the standards are to be met

       c. Evaluating performance involves either concurrent audits to evaluate ongoing care or retrospective audits to evaluate care after patients are discharged

    8. JCAHO mandates open and closed chart reviews by hospital committees on a regularly scheduled basis

    9. Other regulators of health care in the managed care environment include state departments of insurance, National Council for Quality Assurance, and Utilization Review Accreditation Committee as well as JCAHO

   10. Every quality assurance program should have a mechanism for corrective action that addresses unmet outcome criteria

B. Applications to nursing

    1. Nurse managers and leaders play an active role in quality assurance through peer reviews and performance appraisals

    2. A nurse manager should explain to the staff in advance what outcome criteria will be used in evaluation

    3. A nurse manager should work with the staff to implement corrective action for unmet criteria

♦ VI. Continuous quality improvement

A. Key concepts

    1. The total quality management approach involves transforming old quality assurance programs into newer systems that reflect a continuous striving for quality

    2. Quality assurance is being replaced by such terms as *total quality improvement, continuous quality improvement,* and *quality assessment improvement*

    3. These new programs emphasize teamwork over individual performance

    4. In a CQI approach, accountability flows upward from the point of service to administration

       a. CQI encompasses both centralized and decentralized activities that cut across all disciplines involved in patient care

       b. In a CQI program, data are collected and analyzed to address the functioning of an entire system rather than focusing on the individual performance criteria of quality assurance; the functional criteria of CQI, in turn, emphasizes care that is appropriate, effective, and adequate to meet patient care

       c. In CQI, benchmarking is used to select a standard of excellence for a process or procedure; that standard is used to measure related processes or procedures

5. Whereas the focus of care under quality assurance is on controlling quality, the focus of care under CQI is on measuring the appropriateness of care
   a. Both quality control and appropriateness measures are essential
   b. Similar to quality assurance, CQI emphasizes both process and outcome standards

B. Applications to nursing
1. Staff nurses play a fundamental role in a CQI system; the nurse identifies problems, collects data, establishes plans to ensure performance and patient outcomes, and evaluates the plan of care
2. Nurses have an ongoing obligation to establish uniform standards of quality in patient care outcomes

◆ VII. Marketing

A. Key concepts
1. Marketing includes analysis, planning, implementation, and control of a specialized program designed to provide an exchange of goods, services, or values within a specific arena while achieving organizational goals
2. Exchange of goods requires at least two parties, each believing that the other has something of value and each being capable of communication, delivery, and acceptance or rejection of the offer
3. The communication describes the services provided and targets these services to specific population needs
4. Marketing is achieved through a MARKETING PLAN
   a. A successful marketing plan involves the "four Ps": product, price, place, and promotion
   b. Periodic evaluation of the marketing plan allows the organization to meet the changing needs of the target population

B. Applications to nursing
1. Because cost containment and competition have caused health care organizations to promote their services to the public, nursing has become an integral part of each organization's marketing plan
2. Nurses, especially nurse managers, are required to sell themselves as providers of health care to consumers and to the health care organization
3. As health care consumers become more aware of health care options and more selective, nurses at all levels must promote themselves effectively so that the public knows just what they do
4. Nurse managers play a vital role in nursing recruitment and retention and thus can enhance a health care organization's marketability as a provider of quality care

5. A nurse manager also may be responsible for the development and promotion of additional programs to broaden the scope of a health care organization's services, thereby contributing to its profitability

6. Nurse managers may productively utilize nursing staff in community marketing activities involving health promotion, illness prevention, and community safety

♦ VIII. Networking

A. Key concepts

1. Networking refers to the development and use of a professional system for support, guidance, and information to help achieve growth

2. Successful networking requires a positive self-concept, self-awareness, and values clarification

3. A network can include individuals and groups

4. Networking involves role-modeling, power, and politics

5. A person who networks effectively combines the innate tendency to help others with a willingness to use others and, in turn, be used by others in the network

B. Applications to nursing

1. Nurse managers often are members of a staff nurse's network

2. Nurse managers, in turn, have their own network from which to derive support at the unit, department, organizational, and professional levels

3. Nurse managers and leaders use the concepts of power and politics in networking

♦ IX. Mentoring

A. Key concepts

1. Just as networking provides a mechanism for professional support, mentoring provides a mechanism for professional growth

2. Mentoring is a relationship between an experienced nurse (the mentor) and a novice nurse (the protégé); the mentor guides and prepares the protégé for personal and professional advancement

3. Mentoring provides various support mechanisms, including advice, friendship, counseling, and contacts; it paves the way for developing self-confidence and commitment to personal and professional self-actualization, the highest form of motivation

4. Mentoring is different from preceptoring in that preceptoring is a form of staff orientation whereby new nurses learn the tasks and the system from experienced nurses

B. Applications to nursing

1. Mentoring has not been a common phenomenon in nursing

2. Nurses, and women in general, have suffered from a lack of mentors in all areas of professional life, which may contribute to a diminished sense of job satisfaction

3. Mentoring, like networking, is most successful when clear goals and expectations for all parties are communicated and agreed to; a timeline can also be helpful

♦ X. Risk management

A. Key concepts

1. Risk management is a business strategy to reduce or prevent loss and legal action by identifying, analyzing, and evaluating risks and developing plans for reducing the frequency and severity of accidents and injury

2. Health care organizations use risk management to ensure quality control in care delivery and to prevent liability by providing a safe environment and adequate, competent staff members

3. The purpose of risk management in health care is to identify the variables that jeopardize quality care and to correct or minimize them

4. Risk management involves communication, decision making, and change

5. Accountability is the central issue in risk management

6. Successful risk management requires effective communication among all levels of an organization

7. Components of risk management include monitoring devices such as audits, grievances, staffing patterns, and employee and patient INCIDENT REPORTS

B. Applications to nursing

1. A nurse manager is legally responsible for observing, evaluating, and reporting deficiencies in patient care

2. Reporting threats to patient or employee safety is a major responsibility of nurses at all levels; such threats should be documented in the patient's chart and in incident reports

3. A nurse must file an incident report whenever safety or quality is jeopardized; patient injury, staff injury, or medication error must be documented

4. A nurse manager should investigate all incident reports and be alert to deficient care

5. A nurse manager should assure staff nurses that incident reports are used to avoid litigation and ensure quality care, not as a means to discipline or evaluate staff members

6. Educating staff nurses in proper documentation is the nurse manager's responsibility

♦ XI. Stress management

A. Key concepts
1. Stress management involves coping with the body's response to conflict (stress)
2. Stress can be of several sorts: task-based stress, such as work overload; role-based stress, such as conflict between professional and personal roles; institution-based stress, such as understaffing; and personal stress, such as conflict between expectations of performance and perception of that performance
3. Stress is impossible to avoid and is not necessarily harmful
4. Stress can be a positive force (eustress) that adds excitement and challenge to life or a negative force (distress) that impairs effectiveness
5. Accumulation of high stress levels without appropriate management can lead to BURNOUT

B. Applications to nursing
1. A nurse manager should work at the unit, departmental, and organizational levels to minimize or eliminate potential stressors
2. A nurse manager can use a knowledge of conflict resolution, decision making, and networking to develop stress management strategies
3. A nurse manager should teach staff members how to identify sources of stress and eliminate or minimize these stressors; important signs of stress are unusual fatigue, sleepiness, irritability, unexplained sadness, and feelings of loss of control
4. A nurse manager should act as a role model to help staff nurses manage stress
5. A nurse manager can help prevent personal distress and burnout by establishing realistic personal and professional goals and priorities

♦ XII. Team building

A. Key concepts
1. Team building develops a supportive group atmosphere in which members work together effectively toward specific goals
2. Planning, setting goals, and establishing priorities are the first steps in team building
3. GROUP COHESIVENESS is the foundation of team building
4. Communication and group dynamics are essential to team building, group cohesiveness, and team effectiveness
5. The greater the cohesiveness among team members, the greater the group's influence on goal achievement and the greater the group's job satisfaction among individual members
6. Team members are selected for their ability to contribute to the team

SEARCHING THE WEB
Nursing megasites

The nursing megasite produced by the American Nurses Association (www.ajn.org) includes a list of journals that can be reviewed online, including the *Journal of Nursing Administration,* which has helpful articles for nurse leaders and managers.

SpringNet (www.springnet.com) offers links to a wide variety of resources of special interest to nursing students.

B. Applications to nursing

1. A nurse leader or manager should use knowledge of group communication and dynamics to develop a climate that fosters group cohesiveness
2. A nurse leader or manager should assist the team with conflict management and resolution within the team and with other teams
3. A nurse leader or manager should encourage open communication within the team and with other teams

♦ XIII. Leading meetings

A. Key concepts

1. Meetings may be called to discuss and solve problems, ventilate feelings, educate, or share information
2. Planning and organization are essential; an effective meeting should have a set agenda with specific objectives, and it should begin and end on time, allowing for summary and evaluation
3. Leading meetings requires knowledge of power, authority, influence, group dynamics, communication, decision making, and leadership and management styles
4. The person leading the meeting has authority and power and should use a leadership style that enhances the meeting's effectiveness
5. The leader should act as both a leader and a group member in working to achieve the meeting's objectives
6. The environment of the meeting room should be comfortable and allow for group interaction and communication

B. Applications to nursing

1. A nurse leader or manager should participate in meetings to train staff, resolve conflicts, provide motivation, and encourage discussion — which may mean mixing roles as a leader and a group member

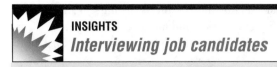

INSIGHTS

Interviewing job candidates

Interviewing is most effective when done in conjunction with a formal application that includes a description of the applicant's skills and knowledge. Interviews should not be conducted casually or without background information; this approach rarely yields enough information for good decision making. During the interview, presenting a simulation of typical problems and asking candidates to describe their responses will provide some insight into how candidates might behave in actual settings. Giving candidates information about the institution early in the application process will help them decide whether that workplace is appropriate for them.

    2. An effective nurse leader or manager uses a knowledge of leadership and management styles, communication, and group dynamics to achieve meeting objectives

    3. A nurse leader or manager uses power to assist group functioning

    4. A nurse leader or manager should communicate the outcome of the meeting to the appropriate personnel and take the necessary steps to implement the outcome at the appropriate level

♦ XIV. Interviewing

A. Key concepts

    1. Interviewing is a step in selecting persons for positions in an organization

    2. Interviewing is a skill that must be learned

    3. Evaluation of information obtained from interviews forms the basis for hiring decisions

    4. Interviewing involves dual communication; the interviewer seeks to gain and evaluate information from the applicant, and the applicant attempts to gather information about the position and the organization

    5. An effective interviewer can solicit information efficiently and gather relevant data

    6. A successful interview requires up-front planning and organization, clear communication about the position and the organization and its goals, and an interest and trust in the applicant (see *Interviewing job candidates*)

    7. Effective interviewing is increasingly important because of legal and ethical constraints present in today's health care workplace

B. Applications to nursing

    1. Nurse managers typically play a significant role in staff recruitment and hiring decisions

2. The organizational structure directly affects the nurse manager's power and authority to interview and hire
3. Conversely, nurse managers often can influence organizational hiring policies
4. A nurse manager communicates information about the health care organization's structure and goals to applicants

POINTS TO REMEMBER

♦ Effective time management is essential to effective managing.

♦ Networking and mentoring can provide important support for personal and professional growth.

♦ Performance appraisals and quality assurance are important parts of a manager's evaluation function.

♦ The emphasis on cost containment in health care delivery has increased the need to market nursing services.

♦ Effectiveness in team building and leading meetings is based on mastering group dynamics.

STUDY QUESTIONS

To evaluate your understanding of this chapter, answer the following questions in the space provided; then compare your responses with the correct answers in appendix B, pages 237 to 244.

1. How is assertiveness related to such skills as time management, risk management, and performance appraisal?_____

_____

_____

2. What is benchmarking and how is it applied in both performance appraisal and continuous quality improvement? _____

_____

_____

3. What two standards are emphasized by quality assurance and continuous quality improvement programs?_____

_____

_____

4. How does a mentor relationship enhance individual motivation? _____

_____

_____

CRITICAL THINKING AND APPLICATION EXERCISES

1. Keep a diary of your activities over a period of several days, identifying amounts of time spent in major tasks. Analyze your record in terms of your abilities to manage time. Did you preestablish amounts of time for significant tasks? Did you establish priorities? What types of unexpected disruptions occurred? How were you able to deal with them? Identify additional actions that you could take to ensure that you use your time most efficiently.

2. Diagram your current network. On a sheet of paper, draw a circle in the center representing yourself. Around a larger circle enclosing the first, list those significant individuals whom you regularly draw on for help and support. On the periphery, draw another circle representing those individuals who could provide support and information, but with whom you less frequently interact. Analyze your diagram. How could you use your network more effectively? How could you more appropriately use the networking resources on the periphery? What can you do to nourish and support your network?

3. Approach a respected nurse leader and ask if she will share information about mentors in her development as a leader. What positions did they occupy? How were they helpful to her? What responsibilities did she have to her mentor? What might this mean for your own development and the identification of potential mentors for you?

9

Budgeting and Resource Allocation

LEARNING OBJECTIVES

After studying this chapter, you should be able to:

♦ Define *budget.*

♦ Describe the common approaches to budgeting.

♦ Identify the major types of budgets.

♦ Describe the nurse manager's role in budgeting.

CHAPTER OVERVIEW

Budgeting involves examining resources, anticipating costs, and predicting gains or shortfalls. Budgets may be incremental or zero-based. Incremental budgeting uses the prior year's budget as a starting point and adds more costs based on projections. The advantage of incremental budgeting is that it is relatively rapid compared to zero-based budgeting and is generally more accepted by staff. Zero-based budgeting requires an institution or a unit to go back to zero in the calculation of the budget for the year, justifying each cost and expenditure. Zero-based budgeting may produce a more precise estimate of costs, but takes much longer and frequently meets with significant staff resistance, as a reduction in budget may result.

♦ I. Introduction

A. Budgeting involves planning and controlling resources that affect the workings of an organization

B. Budgeting is accomplished through a plan called a BUDGET

C. A budget is a detailed outline that describes planned organizational goals and compares them with actual outcomes
1. It attempts to identify problems and determine steps to correct them
2. It provides communication among all levels of managers and their subordinates
3. It shows how resources will be acquired and used over specific intervals
4. It ensures the availability of necessary resources for goal achievement
5. It promotes smooth and efficient organizational operation for goal achievement
6. It acts as a tool for management to make modifications and changes and to project activities necessary for coordinating and achieving organizational goals
7. It helps management control the organization by allocating resources

D. Reimbursement methods include a variety of payment models.
1. Charge per service is payment based on costs plus some margin of profit. Payment is made to the provider after services are rendered, or retrospectively.
2. Cost-based reimbursement, in widespread use during the 1960s and 1970s, is also a retrospective payment model. The payer determines allowable costs and adds some margin of profit.
3. Flat rate reimbursement is a prospective payment model and involves the advance decision of the payer of what treatments or interventions will be covered and at what rate. Medicare utilizes a prospective payment system based on diagnosis-related groups.
4. Capitated payment models are similarly prospective and involve the payer setting a rate for services to a patient over a length of time (months or years).

E. A budget translates organizational goals and outcomes into monetary values to ensure that monies spent (EXPENDITURES) do not exceed monies received (INCOME) within a given period
1. In a budget, money is divided into two categories: income and expenditures
2. Income and expenditures are further divided into subcategories
3. These subcategories may differ according to the service provided by the organization and the approach used for budgeting
4. The desired outcome of any budget is to optimize resources and minimize variance; the optimal use of resources is determined by the accuracy of the initial BUDGET FORECAST and the ongoing evaluation and revision of the budget; profit and loss statements reveal the rela-

tionship of income to expenditure, and how successful the institution has been in accurately predicting both.

F. Two commonly used approaches to budgeting are INCREMENTAL BUDGETING and ZERO-BASED BUDGETING
   1. Incremental budgeting
      a. In this traditional budgeting process, a budget is developed annually based on the expenditures from the previous year
      b. Income and expenditures from the previous year are analyzed and reasons for deviations from the previous budget allocations are evaluated
      c. Projections are made based on the organization's plans and goals, such as salary increases and expansion; these projections usually increase monetary allocations
      d. Dollar figures for income and expenditures are assigned to these projections
      e. The completed budget must be approved by the head of the organization
      f. Anyone with the authority to spend money is required to work within the budget; adjustments may be made but typically are resisted
   2. Zero-based budgeting
      a. This is a participative process based on the assumption that every expenditure must be justified as essential to the organization's function each year; expenditures for the previous year are irrelevant
      b. Each year, the budget begins at zero
      c. Tools called DECISION PACKAGES are compiled and assigned priorities based on the organizational goals and available resources and then implemented
      d. Zero-based budgeting requires more precise planning and allows for more participation than incremental budgeting; it also requires more work and time to complete than incremental budgeting
      e. Zero-based budgeting is frequently used for new services or programs for which financial information is not available

♦ II. Capital expenditure budgets

A. Key concepts
   1. Capital expenditure budgets allocate monies to purchase major equipment or finance major projects, such as expansion or renovation; these monies are called *capital expenditures*
   2. Capital expenditure items usually are major investments that entail long-term cost recovery

3. Capital expenditure budgets typically involve two common criteria: the proposed item must be above a certain specified cost and must have a specified life expectancy, usually several years

4. Capital expenditure budgets require long-range planning

B. Applications to nursing

1. A nurse manager can help anticipate and determine the need for capital expenditures in a health care organization by maintaining close communication with other departments and by keeping current with technological advances and trends

2. A nurse manager must know the budgetary limits on capital expenditures when establishing priorities

3. A nurse manager completes capital expenditure request forms, using information such as depreciation, salvage value, and age of equipment to justify requests

♦ **III. Operating budget**

A. Key concepts

1. Operating budgets allocate monies required to support organizational operation; the two principal operating expenditures are personnel and supplies and equipment

2. An organization's operating budget deals primarily with salaries, supplies, and contractual services

3. Other items, such as materials, work hours, and personnel, can be translated into dollar values as part of the operating budget

B. Applications to nursing

1. Nurse managers play an important role in determining operating budgets

2. With today's emphasis on cost containment in health care, nurse managers are assuming more responsibility for developing operating budgets and controlling operating costs

3. Because of their direct involvement with staffing and scheduling, nurse managers can anticipate needs and justify requests for staffing increases

4. The nurse manager works with staff members to identify changing supply requirements and communicates these changes to superiors

5. The nurse manager monitors the use of equipment and supplies and recommends to the staff ways to minimize costs at the unit level

6. The nurse manager should be aware that health care organizations are hiring hospital management companies to help manage the budgetary pressures of contending with rising costs and reimbursement systems

a. These companies develop strategic plans of 2 to 5 years' duration to ensure cost control, quality control, and competitiveness

SEARCHING THE WEB
Legal and political issues

Nursingnet maintains a forum for discussion of legal and political issues (www.nursingnet.org/boards/legal/index.html). Because budget issues frequently have legal or political implications, having a network of colleagues to discuss these issues with can be very helpful. You can also find out what practices prevail in other parts of the country.

b. These strategic plans are translated into an operating budget that has as a goal the accurate forecasting of fiscal needs, with an emphasis on external events that affect these fiscal needs

Points to remember

◆ Budgeting involves the managerial functions of planning and controlling.

◆ Two common approaches to budgeting are incremental budgeting and zero-based budgeting.

◆ Capital expenditures can include major equipment, expansion, and renovations.

◆ Operating budgets include items such as salaries, supplies, personnel, work hours, and materials.

◆ Nurse managers play a significant role in influencing budgets.

Study questions

To evaluate your understanding of this chapter, answer the following questions in the space provided; then compare your responses with the correct answers in appendix B, pages 237 to 244.

1. What is the desired outcome of any organizational budget?_____

_____

_____

2. How does zero-based budgeting differ from incremental budgeting?_____

_____

_____

3. What are the two principal expenditures in an operating budget? _____

_____

_____

CRITICAL THINKING AND APPLICATION EXERCISES

1. Examine your own budget. Do you use an incremental or zero-based approach to your finances? Do you assume that costs will remain constant and look principally at increases in food prices, rent, and clothing? Do you begin without any assumptions and calculate your expected expenditures on the basis of clearly identified need and cost? What are the advantages and disadvantages of the type of personal budgeting you use?

2. Outline ways in which nurses can help institutions to be more cost-effective. Discuss what the position of the nurse should be with regard to cost containment. What are the risks of not being cost-effective?

3. Speak with the nurse manager about hospital committees that deal with budgets and finance. If possible, arrange to accompany the nurse manager to a committee meeting. Observe what kinds of information are presented and how decisions are made. What input does nursing have, and what role do nurses play on the committee?

10

Staffing and Scheduling

LEARNING OBJECTIVES

After studying this chapter, you should be able to:

♦ Define *staffing*.

♦ Identify the two major types of staffing.

♦ Explain variable and cyclical work schedules.

♦ Discuss the nurse manager's role in each type of staffing.

CHAPTER OVERVIEW

Staffing and scheduling personnel are important managerial tasks. Calculations can either be done by the manager of a particular unit or by central administration. Each method has advantages and disadvantages, but both will reflect the staffing mix, the level of patient acuity, the health care delivery system, and the number of patients to be cared for. Work schedules can be developed for specified time periods (cyclical scheduling) or created on a continuing basis (variable scheduling). Calculation of staffing needs includes identifying the number of required hours of care by the number of productive hours per full-time equivalent staff.

♦ ## I. Introduction

    A. Staffing refers to the number and mix of nursing personnel required for a nursing unit to provide safe, quality, 24-hour patient care

    B. Staffing is determined by
        1. Number and mix of personnel available
        2. PATIENT CENSUS

3. Type of patient care delivery system in use

4. Levels of PATIENT ACUITY

C. Levels of patient acuity are critical to determining the number and type of staff needed to ensure quality care

    1. Various patient classification systems (PCSs) are used to provide data on the level, complexity, and actual costs of care

    2. Some of the PCSs in use include GRASP, Medicus, and APACHE

    3. PCSs can be used to justify the number and qualifications of needed staff

        a. If PCSs are properly managed, nurse managers can objectively quantify nursing in terms of "costing out services"

        b. Costing out services is essential for justifying the need for skilled nursing care and obtaining reimbursement for that care

D. Adequate staffing is essential for quality patient care — the ultimate goal of any health care organization

E. Securing adequate staffing involves developing a work schedule; an effective work schedule enhances nurses' job satisfaction

F. A work schedule can be *cyclical* or *variable*

    1. A CYCLICAL WORK SCHEDULE repeats basic elements over a specified period

        a. Personnel are scheduled to work a specific number of days with specific days off

        b. A cyclical schedule enables personnel to know their schedules in advance and plan accordingly

        c. Cyclical schedules usually are made months in advance

    2. A VARIABLE WORK SCHEDULE changes continually, based on changing staffing needs

        a. Personnel are scheduled according to patient census, patient acuity levels, and level of nursing skill required

        b. Variable schedules use nursing pools, part-time help, and "floats" to supplement the regular staff

G. Staffing structure may be *centralized* or *decentralized,* depending on the organizational structure

♦ **II. Centralized staffing**

A. General information

    1. Centralized staffing allocates personnel by a SCHEDULER, often using a computer

    2. Centralized staffing applies to all nursing units within an organization

    3. It involves consistent, objective, and fair application of organizational policies to all personnel

4. It provides opportunities for cost containment through better use of resources

B. Advantages of centralized staffing
  1. Treats employees fairly and impartially by maintaining consistent staffing policies
  2. Enables preparation of schedules that effectively meet organizational goals
  3. Aids cost containment and time management
  4. Relieves managers from many time-consuming duties
  5. Promotes less frequent special requests from staff for changes in work schedules

C. Disadvantages of centralized staffing
  1. May create or bring out other organizational or managerial problems
  2. Does not address individual workers' abilities, knowledge level, and interests
  3. Does not address variable nursing care needs in particular units

D. Applications to nursing
  1. In a centralized staffing system, the nurse manager typically is responsible for developing a master staffing pattern, clarifying job descriptions, managing personnel, and controlling the personnel budget
  2. The nurse manager must communicate these needs and any changes to the scheduler to ensure adequate staffing

♦ **III. Decentralized staffing**

A. General information
  1. Decentralized staffing allocates personnel at the unit level rather than at the organizational level
  2. Decentralized staffing is congruent with continuous quality improvement; accountability flows from the point of service upward to the administrative levels
  3. With decentralized staffing, a unit manager has the authority and the responsibility to secure adequate personnel for the unit
  4. Decentralized staffing is based on sharing and requires efficient time management; resources may be used less efficiently if time management is inefficient

B. Advantages of decentralized staffing
  1. Enables preparation of individualized schedules based on knowledge of the unit and personnel
  2. Makes the head nurse or nurse manager accountable for staffing decisions

SEARCHING THE WEB
Training for managers

The American Management Association has a Web page (www.amanet.org) listing current journals, seminars, conferences, and other training opportunities of interest to managers.

      3. Enables greater control of activities and rapid schedule adjustments based on changing needs

  C. Disadvantages of decentralized staffing

      1. May be more time-consuming for the nurse manager than centralized staffing

      2. May result in insufficient staffing to meet unforeseen needs

      3. May invite excessive special requests by staff for individualized schedules, making scheduling difficult and time-consuming

  D. Applications to nursing

      1. In a decentralized staffing system, the nurse manager is directly responsible for establishing the personnel allotments and schedules

      2. In decentralized staffing, a nurse manager must be aware of his or her role as the manager and as a group member

      3. Especially in a decentralized staffing system, the nurse manager evaluates the effectiveness of unit staffing and recommends needed changes

      4. Decentralized staffing requires a nurse manager to have excellent time management and communication skills

◆ IV. Calculating staffing needs

  A. Calculation of staffing needs can be done either by the unit or by the central administrative structure

      1. The required hours, or workload volume, is calculated by multiplying the hours of care per patient day by the number of patient days for a particular unit

      2. Total productive hours of full-time equivalent (FTE) staff is calculated as follows: one FTE equal to 2,080 hours of paid work per year, based on a 40-hour week and a 52-week year. The total number of productive work hours (excluding vacation, holiday, and average sick leave utilization) is calculated by subtracting these hours from total FTE hours

      3. The number of FTE needed is calculated by dividing the required hours by the total productive FTE

B. Many variables can interact to produce differences in staffing needs
   1. The type of unit can influence the number of hours per patient day; for example, an intensive care unit requires more hours — and more staff — for the same number of patients as a medical-surgical floor
   2. The staffing mix, including number of unlicensed assistive personnel, can influence staffing needs if responsibility for some elements of care are assigned to others (whose hours must also be calculated)
   3. Collective bargaining contracts may involve agreements about patient acuity and levels of staffing

POINTS TO REMEMBER

♦ Adequate staffing and effective scheduling are essential to providing quality patient care.

♦ Staffing may be centralized or decentralized, depending on the organizational structure.

♦ Work schedules may be cyclical or variable.

♦ The nurse manager plays a major role in centralized or decentralized staffing.

STUDY QUESTIONS

To evaluate your understanding of this chapter, answer the following questions in the space provided; then compare your responses with the correct answers in appendix B, pages 237 to 244.

1. How is staffing determined? _____

   _____

   _____

2. How do patient classification systems help in the professionalization of nursing? _____

   _____

   _____

3. How does decentralized staffing relate to continuous quality improvement? _____

   _____

   _____

CRITICAL THINKING AND APPLICATION EXERCISES

1. Discuss the advantages to management of calculating and assigning staff on a continuing, or variable, basis. What advantages could there be for staff? How would you feel about working on a unit that utilized variable scheduling? How could you plan to adjust to the disadvantages?

2. Talk to a nurse colleague who works in an agency that utilizes cyclical scheduling where work schedules are made out months in advance. What are the advantages of this system? What difficulties has the nurse had with cyclical scheduling when her personal circumstances require a change? How has she dealt with them?

3. Assume that you are the nurse manager on a small unit. Patient acuity requires 3 hours of nursing per patient per day, and you have 1,460 patient-days, for a total workload volume of 4,380 hours. If your nonproductive full time equivalent (FTE) hours (vacation, holiday, and average sick leave) is 26 days per year, leaving you 1,972 productive hours for each full-time equivalent staff member, how many staff will you need? How will the number of FTE hours be affected if the patient acuity required 8.8 hours of care per day?

11

The Changing Health Care Delivery System

LEARNING OBJECTIVES

After studying this chapter, you should be able to:

♦ Discuss how economic change is affecting health care organizations and nursing practice.

♦ Identify the significant demographic changes that are affecting health care delivery and nursing practice.

♦ Identify the changes resulting from the increasing use of advanced technology in health care, and discuss how these changes are affecting nursing practice.

CHAPTER OVERVIEW

Three principal areas of change are having profound impact on the health care delivery system. These include economic changes, demographic changes, and technological changes. Efforts to reduce the cost of health care are being spearheaded by the move to managed care. At the same time, demographic changes are producing a populace that is older, less educated about health care, and more culturally diverse than ever, and technological changes require additional investments in equipment and staff training. Nurses need to be proactively involved in influencing the direction of change for the benefit of patients.

◆ I. Introduction

A. The past decade has been characterized by widespread changes in all aspects of health care that have restructured the health care delivery system and dramatically affected nursing practice

B. The most significant changes — in economics, demographics, and technology — have fragmented health care services

C. Establishing an organized, comprehensive approach to health care delivery is the mandate for the future

D. Nurse leaders and managers can play an essential role in developing this new approach to health care delivery

◆ II. Economic change

A. Key concepts

1. During the past decade, total health care expenditures in the United States have more than doubled

2. This increase has resulted not from improved health care but from inefficient use of resources

3. Federally mandated efforts to reduce expenditures under Medicare legislation have created PROSPECTIVE PAYMENT SYSTEMS and DIAGNOSIS-RELATED GROUPS

4. Increasing consumer demand for quality services despite cost containment has increased competition among health care organizations

5. Private insurers and large corporations also are demanding cost containment and cost-effectiveness

6. Consumers are increasingly demanding excellence and accountability from all health care providers

7. Managed care is increasingly affecting the delivery of health care. Twin goals of managed care include quality patient care and cost-effectiveness, which are promoted through contractual or other agreements that prescribe levels of expenditure per category of patient

B. Applications to nursing

1. Emphasizing cost containment, health care organizations are operating like businesses; consequently, nurses must understand business management concepts and processes

2. Because nursing services account for nearly half the expenditures of health care organizations, nursing departments are pressured to reduce costs while increasing productivity

3. Nurse leaders and managers must become skilled at predicting budgetary and staffing needs to use resources efficiently

4. Nurse leaders and managers must represent their subordinates on committees that determine financial and resource allocation

5. Nurse leaders and managers must stress the need for sufficient nursing staff to ensure quality patient care

6. The economic changes affecting health care challenge nurse leaders and managers to better define nursing practice and to obtain reimbursement for nursing services

7. The shift to for-profit health care may produce ethical dilemmas for nurses if standards of care are perceived as compromised. Nurses should work with colleagues and professional associations to ensure that patients receive appropriate care

8. Nurse leaders and managers are challenged to document and publicize the cost-effectiveness of various types of nursing care, such as care provided by nurse practitioners, nurse midwives, and nurse anesthetists

♦ III. Demographic change

A. Key concepts

1. Changes in the demographic composition of the American population have spurred changes in social, economic, and health care policies and practices

2. The rapidly increasing older population places new burdens on the health care delivery system, such as a demand for home care services and senior day-care centers

3. The significant increase in single-parent families, especially households headed by women, creates new issues for society and the delivery of health care, resulting in increased demand for services such as day care and for more flexible policies such as parental leave for childbirth

4. An increasing minority population expands the need for health care services

5. Certain demographic trends suggest widening poverty in the United States, decreasing the availability of and accessibility to health care services to those who may have great need for such services

B. Applications to nursing

1. The effect of various demographic changes will alter the scope of nursing practice, shifting nursing practice from hospital-based to community-based care and creating more independent and diversified roles that require strong leadership and managerial skills

2. Nursing's holistic approach to health care provides an excellent foundation for addressing the health needs of a changing population

3. Demographic changes will necessitate expanding alternative health care services, creating new opportunities for nursing to expand its role in the health care delivery system

4. Patient needs will direct nursing services toward a HEALTH PROMOTION–disease prevention model of care

5. Nursing practice increasingly will focus on health education and self-care models, which should expand nurses' roles, responsibilities, and power

6. Nurses must become more active in planning and making policy decisions affecting health care

7. In the area of ethics, nurses must be aware that the need for expanded services and the reality of limited resources will force nurses to participate in decisions about who may and may not receive health care services

8. The increase in culturally different immigrants poses challenges in dealing with patients and coworkers; cultural awareness is essential

♦ **IV. Technological change**

A. Key concepts

1. The rapid proliferation of computer information systems is increasing the knowledge base at a phenomenal rate

2. The increasing use of computers in health care organizations is changing the roles of all health care practitioners and improving the efficiency and cost-effectiveness of certain services

3. Computers can provide up-to-the-minute information about patient census, acuity levels, budgetary issues, availability of resources and equipment, and staffing needs; this enables more rapid and more informed decision making at all organizational levels

4. The ever-increasing sophistication and complexity of equipment used in disease diagnosis, treatment, and patient care require ongoing education for all health care practitioners

5. Advanced technology in health care also requires new protocols and procedures for effective management of patient care

B. Applications to nursing

1. The increasing use of computers in health care organizations mandates that all nurses be computer literate

2. Nurse managers find computers invaluable tools for planning, organizing, directing, and evaluating

3. Computers can efficiently perform routine, time-consuming tasks, freeing nurses for more creative and productive activities

4. Computerized information systems provide nurse managers with a constant flow of current information and access to instant communication, which can help speed organizational change

5. Technological advances have created new and highly specialized nursing roles, which, in turn, are changing the lines of communication and decision-making authority within health care organizations

6. Newly specialized nursing roles require ongoing education and retraining for nurses

7. Increasingly sophisticated and complex health care technology often requires nurses to coordinate patient care among numerous health care disciplines

SEARCHING THE WEB

Certification

Information on certification by the American Nurses Association (ANA) can be obtained from the ANA Web site (www.nursingworld.org).
   SpringNet (www.springnet.com) offers a wealth of information on NCLEX and other certification issues.

♦ V. Health care reform

A. Key concepts

1. The American Nurses Association (ANA) and other professional associations have called for reform of the health care delivery system
2. Included in the proposals are:
   a. Restructuring to enhance consumer access
   b. Identification of a standard health care package to be available to all citizens
   c. Public and private plans to deliver at least the standard health care package
   d. A phase-in period to begin with pregnancy and child coverage
   e. Decreasing costs through the use of managed care
   f. Case management of health care
   g. Long-term care coverage
   h. Insurance reform
   i. System review and evaluation on a continuing basis

B. Implications for nurses

1. Health care reform will require a longer period than at first envisioned
2. Nurses can advocate for elements of the ANA proposal, including greater access for vulnerable groups, including children and pregnant women
3. Nurses can work politically with other groups to bring forward new legislative proposals that incrementally introduce health care reform

POINTS TO REMEMBER

♦ Significant changes in economics, demographics, and technology are profoundly affecting health care delivery and nursing practice.

♦ Economic changes primarily involve cost containment and cost-effectiveness.

♦ Various demographic changes, such as the increasing number of older and minority populations and single-family households, will alter the scope of nursing practice.

♦ Technological changes—specifically, the use of computers and advanced equipment in health care delivery—are altering nurses' decision-making responsibilities and communication lines.

STUDY QUESTIONS

To evaluate your understanding of this chapter, answer the following questions in the space provided; then compare your responses with the correct answers in appendix B, pages 237 to 244.

1. How have economic changes affected the health care delivery system?

_____

_____

2. How have demographic changes affected the scope of nursing practice?

_____

_____

3. What elements are included in the proposal for health care reform by the American Nurses' Association? _____

_____

_____

CRITICAL THINKING AND APPLICATION EXERCISES

1. Obtain copies of the census information for your county for the last two censuses. Describe the changes that have occurred in age distributions. What are the changes in cultural affiliation? What impact do you believe these changes have had on the delivery of health care in your environment?

2. One rationale for the institution of a national health care service is that it would drastically change the relationship of insurers to patients. Because a certain level of care would be mandated under private and public health plans, all patients would be eligible for certain fully covered benefits. Discuss the debate of this proposal. What disadvantages could there be in having the state or national government monitoring health care and reimbursement?

12

Issues in Nursing Leadership and Management

LEARNING OBJECTIVES

After studying this chapter, you should be able to:

♦ Describe the collective bargaining process.

♦ Describe the steps involved in a grievance procedure.

♦ Define the role a budget plays in cost containment.

♦ Define *staffing*.

CHAPTER OVERVIEW

Current issues in nursing leadership and management include collective bargaining, dealing with employee grievances, promoting cost containment, and avoiding inadequate staffing. Employee grievances can result from violations of the collective bargaining agreement, violations of federal or state laws, discontinuation of past standard practices, health and safety violations, or violations of the employer's own policies or regulations. Cost containment and staffing decisions must be made in such a manner as not to compromise patient care.

♦ I. Introduction

A. Consumers, government, and third-party payers demand quality health care in a safe environment

B. In today's atmosphere of cost containment, quality care must also be cost-effective care

C. Nurses are becoming increasingly accountable for ensuring quality care

D. Health care organizations are accountable for providing an environment that promotes quality care

E. The quality of care can be monitored through a quality control program

F. Employee grievances, collective bargaining, cost containment, and staffing are important components of a quality control program

G. Quality control of nursing care at the unit level is primarily the nurse manager's responsibility

H. Health care organizations that do not meet employee demands for an effective and safe work environment may become the target of COLLECTIVE BARGAINING efforts to improve working conditions

I. Other elements that may be covered by collective bargaining agreements and that affect health care delivery include the identification of nursing responsibilities under managed care and the emergence of advance nursing practice roles

◆ II. Collective bargaining

A. Key concepts
1. Collective bargaining provides a means for workers and management to meet and solve conflicts about working conditions, wages, work load, hours, and various GRIEVANCES
2. Collective bargaining is a legal process carried out through a union or other labor organization
3. Collective bargaining results in a labor agreement or contract that specifies the rights and responsibilities of both workers and management
4. An increasing number of health care institutions are participating in collective bargaining
5. The National Labor Relations Act of 1935 (also known as the Wagner Act) established the right of workers to join unions and created the National Labor Relations Board (NLRB), whose purpose is to enforce the act and curb unfair labor practices
   a. In 1967, the NLRB was given jurisdiction over proprietary hospitals and nursing homes; in 1975, the NLRB was given jurisdiction over nonprofit hospitals
   b. The NLRB resolves disputes between an employer and a bargaining unit; if an agreement is not reached but both parties are unwilling to compromise, the bargaining unit may decide to strike in hopes of forcing the employer to make concessions

6. The American Nurses Association (ANA) established an Economic Security Program in 1946, which established national salary guidelines for nurses
7. Health care workers have become increasingly involved in unions, and nurses have begun to organize and strike through state nurses' groups
8. In most instances, health care workers form or join unions to help gain fair pay, job security, and good working conditions
9. Nurses tend to form or join unions for economic and professional reasons, typically related to frustration concerning a perceived lack of control over their practice and lack of input into decision making in health care organizations
10. In health care organizations, a notice to strike must be given 10 days before the strike; a request for any change in the collective bargaining agreement requires 90 days' written notice (compared with the 60 days' notice required in other industries)
11. Interest-based bargaining, in which both parties address issues on the basis of interests rather than entrenched, preestablished positions, is a promising alternative to traditional positional negotiations (see *Interest-based bargaining*)

B. Applications to nursing
1. Nurses should be aware of and clarify their own values regarding collective bargaining and strikes when choosing a workplace
2. Nurses also need to protect themselves from unfair management practices
3. Nurses working in a health care organization with a collective bargaining agreement should obtain and study a copy of the collective bargaining contract, which specifies conditions of employment, such as salaries, workload, fringe benefits, and advancement opportunities as well as specific procedures for filing grievances regarding various issues
4. Collective bargaining contracts establish *nurse practice committees,* which allow employees to become involved in health care decisions
5. A nurse manager should review past positions taken by both the union and management on contract negotiations, grievances, and decisions to strike; this information can help the nurse manager identify and address key issues before they become problematic
6. In a health care organization that displays minimal concern for employee satisfaction, a nurse leader may become instrumental in lobbying for a collective bargaining agreement

♦ III. Employee grievances

A. Key concepts
1. A labor agreement or contract typically specifies a detailed procedure for filing employee grievances

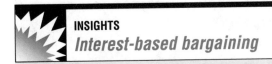

INSIGHTS

Interest-based bargaining

When traditional negotiations prove unsuccessful, one way to break out of entrenched positional bargaining is to move to interest-based bargaining. Under this type of bargaining, all members of the bargaining team, along with administration, go through training to learn to present concerns and issues as interests and to learn to articulate not only their own interests, but those of the other side as well. Choices that can be made in isolation, in collaboration, or by the other side are examined. The purpose is to find a solution that recognizes the interests of workers and management.

 2. Grievances generally fall into two categories: unfair labor practices or violations of a contract, precedent, or past practice

 3. A grievance may represent a violation of the contract or a misunderstanding of the contract, or it may be a means of expressing employee dissatisfaction

 4. The grievance procedure typically begins with an informal discussion between the employee and the manager

 5. If informal communication fails to resolve the issue, the next step is formal communication (a written appeal), followed by a meeting of the employee, a management representative, and a union representative

 6. If the grievance remains unresolved, it goes to a neutral third party for ARBITRATION

 7. Employees may also make complaints about sexual harassment or discrimination, which are subject to regulation outside the collective bargaining arena

B. Applications to nursing

 1. Nurses who participate in a grievance procedure need to learn and use the concepts of conflict resolution, communication, decision making, and group dynamics

 2. When initiating a grievance procedure, the nurse should know and use the formal channels of oral and written communication

 3. A thorough analysis of the grievance along with an exploration of similar instances in the past should guide the nurse manager in decision making

 4. Resolution of a grievance should result in a *win-win solution* for the nurse and nursing management; this will create a constructive climate for future grievance procedures

 5. A contract provides a solution to employee grievances; the nurse manager must base decisions on contract stipulations, rather than on personal power or authority (see *Legitimate grievances,* page 112)

Legitimate grievances

Examples of five categories of legitimate employee grievances are shown below.

Contract violations

Your employment contract is binding on you *and* your employer. If your employer violates the contract, you have a valid grievance. In the following examples, assume that the contract prohibits the employer action described:
• You're performing the charge nurse's job 2 or 3 days a week but are still receiving the same pay as other staff nurses.
• You've had to work undesirable shifts or on Sundays more often than other nurses.
• Your supervisor doesn't post time schedules in advance.
• Your employer discharges you without just cause.

Federal and state law violations

Any action by your employer that violates a federal or state law would be the basis for a grievance, even if your contract permits the action. For example:
• A female nurse receives less pay for performing the same work as a male nurse.
• You don't receive overtime pay that you're entitled to.
• Your employer doesn't promote you because of your race.

Past practice violations

A past practice—one that's been accepted by both parties over an extended period and is suddenly discontinued by the employer without notification—may be the basis for a grievance. For example:
• Your employer charges you for breaking equipment when others haven't been charged.
• Your employer revokes parking lot privileges.
• Your employer eliminates a rotation system for float assignments.
   A past practice violation can occur even if the past practice isn't specified in the contract. If the practice violates the contract, either party can demand that the contract be enforced. If the practice is unsafe, an arbitrator may simply abolish it.

Health and safety violations

Grievances in this category most often involve working conditions that an employer is responsible for, even if the contract doesn't cover the specific complaint. For example:
• You're required to hold patients during X-rays.
• You have no hand-washing facilities near patient rooms.

Employer policy violations

Your employer can't violate its own rules without being guilty of a grievance, even though it can change the rules unilaterally. For example:
• You haven't received a performance evaluation in 2 years, although your employee handbook states that such evaluations will be done annually.
• Your employer assigns you a vacation period without your consent, contrary to personnel policies.

♦ IV. Cost containment

A. Key concepts

1. The economic changes in health care over the past decade have created a climate of competition for funding and resources among health care organizations

2. Cost containment involves minimizing expenditures and maximizing efficiency; at the unit level, nurses are pressured to curtail cost while increasing efficiency

3. Because nursing care is not a separate reimbursable item but is instead included in the patient's room rate, cost containment of nursing at the unit level is difficult

4. Identifying clear, measurable nursing goals — such as those in a management-by-objectives (MBO) system — along with various cost accounting measures may help contain nursing expenditures
   a. MBO focuses on maximizing the efficiency and quality of care
   b. Cost accounting focuses on critically analyzing expenses with an eye toward improving the use of resources

5. Gainsharing — giving employees a financial incentive by allowing them to share in the institution's profits — is one way of making employees more conscious of measures to improve efficiency and reduce waste

6. Cost containment requires managerial planning and evaluation through a budget, which serves as a plan for using resources and an evaluation of how the resources have been used

B. Applications to nursing

1. Nurse leaders and managers should understand their health care organization's formal structure, philosophy, and objectives — all of which influence the operating budget

2. The budget outlines a way for a nurse manager to achieve individual and organizational goals; meeting these goals promotes job satisfaction

3. Resource use is enhanced by a knowledge of economic, demographic, and technological changes in health care, which helps the nurse manager predict operating costs

4. Involving staff nurses in cost containment by sharing budget information and budgetary goals is a wise nursing management strategy

5. Encouraging staff participation in cost containment helps motivate staff nurses to work more efficiently and productively, especially when the budget allows for staff education, research, and innovation in care

SEARCHING THE WEB
State nursing associations

Information on state nursing associations can be accessed from the American Nurses Association Web site (www.nursingworld.org/snas). These Web pages provide updates on meetings, conferences, collective bargaining issues, and political actions at the state level.

♦ V. Inadequate staffing

A. Key concepts
1. Staffing involves determining the number and mix of nurses needed on a unit to provide quality patient care 24 hours a day
2. With today's emphasis on cost containment in health care, staffing must be cost-effective, yet sufficient to meet patient needs
3. Staffing and work schedules greatly affect nurses' job satisfaction and productivity, which ultimately affects patient care
4. Insufficient or ineffective staffing or scheduling can cause discontent, frustration, stress, poor morale, increased turnover, and absenteeism

B. Applications to nursing
1. The nurse manager must be able to provide adequate staffing, working within the constraints of cost containment
2. The nurse manager also has an ethical and legal responsibility to provide sufficient staffing to ensure patient safety
3. Unsafe staffing practices, such as moving nurses to unfamiliar units or making nurses work double shifts, may create ethical or legal dilemmas for the nurse manager; for example, insufficient staffing may provide appropriate grounds for a patient to sue for neglect
4. A nurse manager should involve staff nurses in planning schedules whenever possible; this can help increase motivation and decrease absenteeism
5. A nurse manager should never manipulate staffing schedules to punish employees; this is an unfair use of power
6. If staff nurses are unionized, the nurse manager must consider any staffing patterns mandated by the labor contract
7. In organizations that use centralized staffing systems, nurse leaders and managers should participate in staffing review committees to communicate staffing needs to higher management
8. Decentralized staffing takes more time for a nurse manager; the nurse manager can save time by basing the staffing plan on an accepted staffing standard such as the ANA's "Nursing Staff Requirements for In-Patient Health Care Services"

9. When reductions in workforce must be made, the nurse manager can do much to alleviate concern and avoid rumor and misunderstanding by communicating promptly and accurately to staff

POINTS TO REMEMBER

♦ With today's emphasis on cost containment, quality care also must be cost-effective care.

♦ Health care organizations, unlike other industries, must give 90 days' written notice before changes can be made in a labor contract.

♦ A grievance may represent a violation of the labor contract or a misinterpretation of it, or it may be a means of expressing employee dissatisfaction.

♦ Cost containment poses a significant challenge to nurses at all levels of a health care organization.

♦ Inadequate staffing patterns may create legal and ethical dilemmas for a nurse manager.

STUDY QUESTIONS

To evaluate your understanding of this chapter, answer the following questions in the space provided; then compare your responses with the correct answers in appendix B, pages 237 to 244.

1. What role does the National Labor Relations Board play in collective bargaining? _____

_____

_____

2. How many days' notice must a health care organization receive before employees can strike? _____

_____

_____

3. How would the practice of gainsharing affect cost containment at the unit level? _____

_____

_____

4. How might inadequate staffing affect a nurse's job satisfaction and productivity? _____

_____

_____

CRITICAL THINKING AND APPLICATION EXERCISES

1. Talk with the Human Resources Director at a local health care agency about the most frequent types of employee grievances. What could have been done to avoid a grievance being filed? Could the manager have taken action earlier to deal with the situation?

2. Look in the employee lounge or staff briefing area of a local hospital. Are there Occupational Safety and Health Organization or other safety notices posted? What do they advise staff to do with concerns? Are there notices posted for collective bargaining agents? What issues do they concern? How can being aware of the issues and focuses of regulatory groups and collective bargaining entities help a nurse manager deal more proactively with employee concerns?

3. Imagine that you are the manager on a unit that will undergo reorganization and a reduction in workforce. How will you communicate this to your staff? What questions do you expect that they will have? How will you work with the staff remaining to deal with continuing concerns about job security?

Introduction to Nursing Research

LEARNING OBJECTIVES

After studying this chapter, you should be able to:

♦ Describe the goals of nursing research.

♦ Identify the sources of nursing knowledge.

♦ Discuss the evolution of nursing research over the last century and the implications for future nursing research.

♦ List the major steps in performing research.

♦ Identify the responsibilities that nurses, depending on their education, may be expected to assume in research.

CHAPTER OVERVIEW

This chapter contains an introduction and an overview of some tenets related to nursing research. It also provides a historical perspective on nursing research, the steps required to conduct research, and the nurse's responsibilities in research.

♦ **I. Overview of nursing research**

    A. The primary goal of nursing RESEARCH is to develop a specialized, scientifically based body of knowledge unique to nursing

    B. Nursing research has other goals as well
       1. Developing and testing nursing theories
       2. Providing an understanding of phenomena related to nursing

  3. Fostering professional commitment and accountability
  4. Helping nurses to make informed decisions in the delivery of pa-
     tient care
  5. Validating the effectiveness of particular nursing measures
  6. Helping to document nursing's unique role in health care delivery
  7. Improving the quality of care and care delivery
  8. Providing a link between theory and practice
  9. Advancing nursing as a profession

C. Nursing research that uses the *scientific method* is one of the primary
   sources of nursing knowledge

D. The scientific method is a systematic approach
  1. It attempts to control variables and biases
  2. It uses EMPIRICAL EVIDENCE to develop generalizable results

E. Researchers use the scientific method primarily for five tasks
  1. Describing phenomena
  2. Exploring the relationships among phenomena
  3. Explaining phenomena and increasing understanding
  4. Predicting the causes of and relationships among phenomena
  5. Controlling phenomena

F. Basing nursing research on the scientific method is limiting
  1. Every research study has flaws
  2. No single study proves or disproves a hypothesis
  3. Ethical issues can constrain researchers
  4. Holistic studies of humans are difficult
  5. Adequate control is hard to maintain in a study

G. Nursing knowledge also relies on six other sources
  1. Tradition
  2. Authority
  3. Intuition
  4. Trial and error
  5. Personal experience
  6. Logical reasoning (INDUCTIVE or DEDUCTIVE)

H. Nursing research can be basic or applied
  1. *Basic* research
     a. Undertaken to advance knowledge in a given area
     b. Helps the researcher to understand relationships among phenomena
  2. *Applied* research
     a. Undertaken to remedy a particular problem or modify a situation
     b. Helps the researcher to make decisions or evaluate techniques

I. Nursing research can be quantitative or qualitative
  1. Quantitative research examines specific phenomena
  2. Qualitative research explores human experiences as they are lived

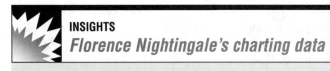

INSIGHTS

Florence Nightingale's charting data

Florence Nightingale collected mortality data for the British soldiers in the Crimean War. To illustrate the significance of the data, she created charts that gave a visual presentation of the mortality rates of the soldiers compared with their counterparts in England. She used the data to help bring about changes and lower mortality rates.

◆ **II. Historical perspective**

A. 1850 to 1949

1. Attempts at nursing research began in the 1850s with Florence Nightingale

a. She emphasized the importance of systematic observation, data collection, environmental factors, and statistical analyses

b. Nightingale's research led to attitudinal and organizational changes for nursing and society at large (see *Florence Nightingale's charting data*)

2. Research in the early 1900s focused mainly on nursing education; however, case studies on nursing interventions were also conducted in the late 1920s and 1930s, the results of which were published in the *American Journal of Nursing*

3. The Goldmark Report of 1923, a comprehensive study of nursing education, recommended reorganizing the nursing education system and incorporating it into the university setting

4. The Brown Report of 1948, which recommended further analysis of nursing functions and nurses' relationships with patients, led to a system for classifying and accrediting nursing schools

B. 1950 to 1959

1. During the 1950s, research mainly studied nursing activities

2. Research courses were introduced into baccalaureate-degree nursing programs, and more research courses were added at the master's-degree level

3. *Nursing Research* began publication in 1952

4. The American Nurses' Foundation was chartered in 1955 to help the growing number of nurses with advanced education to fund and conduct nursing research

5. The first nursing unit for clinical practice–oriented research was established in 1957 at the Walter Reed Army Institute of Research

C. 1960 to 1969

1. During the 1960s, research began to focus on clinical studies

    2. The American Nurses Association (ANA) sponsored the first nursing research conference aimed at disseminating research findings in 1965

    3. In 1968, nursing archives for historical research were established at Boston University

    4. Nursing studies began to explore theoretical and conceptual frameworks as a basis for practice

D. 1970 to 1979

    1. During the 1970s, research focused mainly on improving patient care

    2. The ANA established the Commission on Nursing Research in 1972 to facilitate the exchange of ideas among researchers and to recognize excellence in research

    3. Additional research journals, such as *Advances in Nursing Science* (1978), *Research in Nursing and Health* (1978), and *Western Journal of Nursing Research* (1979), began publication

    4. The National League for Nursing began to consider research a necessary component in the accreditation of nursing education programs

E. 1980 to 1989

    1. In the 1980s, interest in qualitative nursing research grew

    2. The number of doctoral-level nursing programs and students increased, resulting in increased research

    3. The ANA created the Center for Research for Nursing in 1983 to develop reliable data for the profession

    4. The National Center for Nursing Research was established within the National Institutes of Health in 1985, putting nursing research into the mainstream of health research activities

F. 1990 to the present

    1. The 1990s have seen an increase in integrative reviews, meta-analyses, and more sophisticated model-testing research

    2. The Agency for Health Care Policy and Research of the U.S. Department of Health and Human Services' Public Health Service developed clinical practice guidelines based on research

    3. In 1993, the National Center for Nursing Research was renamed the National Institute for Nursing Research, putting nursing research on the same level as other health-related research

    4. Sigma Theta Tau established the Virginia Henderson International Nursing Library, an electronic library making information accessible to researchers worldwide

    5. The first electronic nursing journal, the *Online Journal of Knowledge Synthesis for Nursing,* was established in 1993 and publishes critical reviews of research literature

G. Priorities for future nursing research

    1. Promoting health and preventing illness among all groups

    2. Preventing behaviorally and environmentally induced health problems

3. Testing community-based nursing models
4. Ensuring the effectiveness of nursing interventions in human immunodeficiency virus infection and acquired immunodeficiency syndrome
5. Assessing approaches for remediating cognitive impairment
6. Evaluating approaches to living with chronic illness
7. Identifying biobehavioral factors related to immunocompetence
8. Documenting the effectiveness of health care services
9. Expanding health service research focused on outcomes
10. Determining the cost-effectiveness of patient care

♦ III. Steps in performing research

A. General information
1. A research study typically follows a sequence of steps
2. At each step, the researcher makes decisions that affect the study
3. Before conducting a major research study, the researcher may perform a PILOT STUDY, which minimizes the possibility of encountering serious difficulties in the major study and obtains information for improving the major study

B. Research problem selection (see chapter 15)
1. The researcher selects a problem that clarifies the focus of the study
2. The focus moves from a general topic to a specific problem
3. The researcher culminates by formulating a PURPOSE STATEMENT

C. Literature review (see chapter 16)
1. The researcher uses related literature to examine knowledge to date
2. The literature must be relevant to the concepts (variables) identified in the purpose statement
3. The review helps direct the researcher in designing the study and interpreting the results

D. Conceptual and theoretical frameworks (see chapter 17)
1. These provide structure and link components
2. They provide a context within which the researcher can interpret the study's results

E. Variables, hypotheses, and research questions (see chapter 18)
1. The researcher predicts the study's outcome based on the relationship among the variables
2. When a researcher is interested in exploring a phenomenon, a research question rather than a hypothesis may be used
3. The researcher must specify how the variables are viewed and how they will be measured

F. Research designs (see chapter 19)
1. The design provides guidelines with which the researcher tests the hypotheses

2. It directs the selection of the POPULATION, sampling technique, and plan for the researcher's data collection and analysis

G. Sampling techniques (see chapter 20)
1. These establish the criteria that the researcher uses to include subjects
2. They outline how the subjects will be selected
3. The human rights of the study participants are protected

H. Data collection methods and measurement techniques (see chapter 21)
1. The collected data provide the researcher with the information needed to answer the research question
2. How the data are collected can influence the study's outcome
3. Data should be evaluated according to specific techniques

I. Data analysis (see chapter 22)
1. The researcher consolidates and organizes the data to produce findings that can be interpreted
2. Analysis involves descriptive and statistical techniques, or logical explanations

J. Interpretation, communication, and use of research findings (see chapter 23)
1. The researcher draws conclusions from the data and makes recommendations for action or further study
2. The researcher relates the findings to previous research and to the conceptual or theoretical framework
3. The researcher disseminates the study's findings for use

♦ IV. Nurses' responsibilities in research

A. General information
1. Any nurse can participate in research and use its findings
2. In 1981, the ANA developed guidelines to help nursing educators prepare nurses for research, according to their academic level
3. As educational preparation increases, the researcher's sophistication also increases
4. Nurses at all academic and professional levels need to critique previously conducted and newly proposed research

B. Responsibilities of graduates from associate-degree nursing programs
1. Demonstrate awareness of the value of research
2. Assist in identifying problem areas and collecting data

C. Responsibilities of graduates from baccalaureate-degree nursing programs
1. Read, interpret, and evaluate research reports
2. Apply research findings to nursing practice
3. Identify nursing problems for investigation
4. Share research findings with peers
5. Participate in research projects

SEARCHING THE WEB
Knowledge synthesis

Get more information on the *Online Journal of Knowledge Synthesis for Nursing* at www.stti.iupui.edu/publications/journal.

D. Responsibilities of graduates from master's-degree nursing programs
1. Analyze and reformulate nursing problems so that they can be tested
2. Provide nursing expertise to help identify research problems and direct research
3. Conduct scientific investigations
4. Collaborate, consult, and assist with others in research projects and in applying findings

E. Responsibilities of graduates from doctoral-degree nursing programs
1. Appraise, design, and conduct nursing research
2. Develop theoretical explanations of nursing phenomena
3. Develop methods of scientific inquiry
4. Use analytical and empirical methods to modify or extend knowledge
5. Provide leadership in promoting nursing research

POINTS TO REMEMBER

♦ Nursing research is essential for developing a scientific knowledge base and for advancing nursing as a profession.

♦ Nursing knowledge is derived from the scientific method, tradition, authority, intuition, trial and error, personal experience, and logical reasoning.

♦ Nursing research may be basic or applied, quantitative or qualitative.

♦ Nursing research has been shaped by key historical events.

♦ Research includes sequential steps that provide order and control.

♦ Every nurse, regardless of educational level, has certain responsibilities in the research process.

STUDY QUESTIONS

To evaluate your understanding of this chapter, answer the following questions in the space provided; compare your responses with the correct answers in appendix B, pages 237 to 244.

1. What is the primary goal of nursing research? _____

_____

_____

2. What is the difference between basic research and applied research?

_____

_____

3. What contributions did Florence Nightingale make to nursing research?

_____

_____

4. Why might a researcher conduct a pilot study? _____

_____

_____

5. What is the responsibility of all nurses, regardless of academic or professional level, in research?_____

_____

_____

CRITICAL THINKING AND APPLICATION EXERCISES

1. Consider how the following sources of nursing knowledge are used in your practice:

   a. Tradition

   b. Authority

   c. Intuition

   d. Trial and error

   e. Personal experience

   f. Logical reasoning

   g. Research

2. Describe a nursing intervention that is based on research.

3. Find an article reporting a nursing research study. Determine if the research is basic or applied.

4. Read a quantitative research article and a qualitative research article. How are they alike? How are they different?

Ethical Considerations in Nursing Research

CHAPTER OVERVIEW

This chapter identifies the ethical concerns and historical events affecting research. Selected professional guidelines and ethical codes along with the federal guidelines related to conducting ethical research are discussed. The human rights that require protection and the elements of informed consent are outlined. Pertinent questions to consider when critiquing the ethical aspects of a research study are listed.

♦ I. Introduction

A. Nursing research must be ethical in its development and implementation to protect human subjects without compromising the quality of the research

B. Ethics in nursing research involves applying those principles and actions mandated by professional, legal, and social rules to protect human subjects

C. Ethical actions taken by researchers should include four components
 1. Protecting the rights of subjects
 2. Ensuring that a study's potential benefits outweigh its risks to the subjects
 3. Submitting the proposed study for institutional review
 4. Obtaining an INFORMED CONSENT from each subject

♦ II. Historical events affecting ethical research

A. General information
 1. Unethical experiments and mistreatment of human research subjects in early studies prompted the need for ethical conduct in research and led to the development of professional guidelines and ethical codes
 2. Experimental studies noted for unethical treatment of human subjects include Nazi medical experiments, the Tuskegee syphilis study, the Jewish Chronic Disease Hospital study, and the Willowbrook hepatitis study

B. Nazi medical experiments
 1. Conducted from 1933 to 1945 by the Third Reich in Europe
 2. Included euthanasia, sterilization, and numerous medical experiments, such as exposing subjects to high altitudes, freezing temperatures, diseases, and untested drugs
 3. Based the selection of subjects on political or religious grounds (prisoners of war, Jews)
 4. Allowed no opportunity for subjects to refuse participation
 5. Performed to generate knowledge and eliminate "inferior" people and promote "racial purity"

C. Tuskegee syphilis study
 1. Performed in Tuskegee, Alabama, from 1932 to 1972 under the supervision of the U.S. Public Health Service
 2. Conducted to determine the course of syphilis in adult black males
 3. Withheld from the subjects knowledge about the availability of penicillin after it proved to be an effective treatment

4. Also withheld information about the purpose of the research

D. Jewish Chronic Disease Hospital study
1. Conducted in 1963 in Brooklyn, New York
2. Involved the injection of live cancer cells into 22 patients to determine their rejection responses
3. Conducted without the informed consent of the subjects, knowledge of the subjects' physicians, or approval from the hospital research committee

E. Willowbrook hepatitis study
1. Conducted during the 1960s and 1970s in Willowbrook, New York
2. Used institutionalized, mentally impaired children as subjects
3. Inoculated groups of newly institutionalized children with hepatitis viruses to evaluate their responses
4. Forced parents to consent by allowing admissions to the research ward only

♦ III. Professional guidelines and codes

A. General information
1. Abuse of human subjects by unethical researchers directly influenced the development of ethical codes and guidelines
2. Codes and guidelines developed by professional groups to govern ethical behavior and conduct are difficult to formulate because definitions of "right" and "wrong" are typically vague and subjective
3. Researchers must consider ethical guidelines continuously during a study to ensure that research is conducted ethically (see *Ethical aspects of research,* page 128)

B. The Nuremberg Code
1. Developed in 1949 as a result of unethical experimentation spotlighted during Nazi criminal trials
2. Was the first international effort to create formal standards involving human research subjects
3. Included guidelines for voluntary consent, subjects' protection from harmful experiments, subjects' right to withdraw from a study, grounds for discontinuing a study, the need for balance between potential risks and potential benefits in a study, and the researcher's necessary qualifications

C. The Declaration of Helsinki
1. Adopted in 1964 and revised in 1975 by the World Medical Association
2. Based on the Nuremberg Code
3. Differentiated therapeutic research, such as research conducted to explore the beneficial effects of a new treatment, from nontherapeutic research aimed toward building a knowledge base

CHECKLIST

Ethical aspects of research

Use the following questions to critique the ethical aspects of a research study.

	Yes	No
• Was the research approved by an institutional review board or a similar ethical committee?	☐	☐
• Was the researcher qualified to conduct the study?	☐	☐
• Did the study's potential benefits for subjects outweigh the risks?	☐	☐
• Did the researcher take measures to prevent or minimize psychological and physical harm or discomfort to the subjects?	☐	☐
• Were the subjects recruited without coercion?	☐	☐
• Were the subjects told about the potential benefits and risks associated with participation?	☐	☐
• Did the researcher disclose sources of funding?	☐	☐
• Were the study's purposes and procedures fully explained in advance to the subjects?	☐	☐
• Did the researcher obtain informed consent from all participating subjects?	☐	☐
• Did all subjects have an opportunity to decline participation before and during the study?	☐	☐
• If vulnerable subjects were used, was their inclusion necessary?	☐	☐
• Was each subject's right to privacy and anonymity protected?	☐	☐
• Did the researcher maintain objectivity when reporting the findings?	☐	☐
• Did the researcher credit others who assisted with the study?	☐	☐

4. Identified the importance of qualifying the type of research (therapeutic or nontherapeutic) when explaining potential benefits and risks to prospective subjects
5. Stated that subjects must be informed of the personal risks and potential benefits before agreeing to participate
6. Emphasized the importance of subjects' written consent

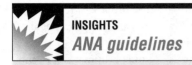

INSIGHTS
ANA guidelines

As the professional organization for nurses, the American Nurses Association (ANA) sets standards and develops guidelines for practice. Six guidelines and their implementation in clinical and other research have been outlined by the association.

D. American Nurses Association Human Rights Guidelines
  1. Developed in 1968 and revised in 1975 and 1985 as specific guidelines for nursing research
  2. Addressed ethical and practical issues related to clinical research
  3. Outlined the rights of nurses to perform research and to gather information and knowledge necessary to complete research studies
  4. Identified the rights of subjects and nurses involved in research (see *ANA guidelines*)

♦ **IV. Federal ethical research guidelines**

A. General information
  1. The Department of Health, Education, and Welfare proposed the first set of regulations for protecting human subjects in 1973
  2. Strict regulations for research involving human subjects were published in May 1974, along with additional regulations for vulnerable populations, such as terminally ill and mentally impaired individuals, children, and persons confined to institutions

B. The Belmont Report
  1. Presented in 1979 by the National Commission for the Protection of Human Subjects
  2. Provided the basis for the development of various protective procedures, such as informed consent
  3. Identified three ethical principles relevant to research
    a. Respect
    b. Beneficence
    c. Justice

C. The National Research Act
  1. The National Research Act of 1974 mandated the use of an INSTITUTIONAL REVIEW BOARD (IRB) for any organization receiving federal funding and performing research with human subjects
  2. IRBs review research studies, ensure the protection of subjects' rights, and report noncompliance by researchers

3. IRBs are authorized to approve or disapprove proposals, require modifications, or suspend the approval of research; approval of all proposals must meet federal guidelines
4. Studies demonstrating no apparent risk or only minimal risk to subjects may receive a brief review; studies demonstrating a higher risk receive a full IRB review
5. A study must receive some form of IRB approval before the researcher can initiate it

◆ V. Protection of human rights

A. General information
1. Human rights are demands or privileges to which a person is entitled
2. The main purpose of professional guidelines and ethical codes is to protect human rights
3. In any study, the researcher must weigh potential benefits and risks
4. VULNERABLE SUBJECTS, such as hospitalized patients, children, prisoners, or the mentally incompetent, require additional protection of their human rights
5. Human rights that require protection include the rights to self-determination, privacy, ANONYMITY or CONFIDENTIALITY, fair treatment, and protection from harm

B. Right to self-determination
1. The right to self-determination is a person's right to act independently and make individual decisions
2. This right is protected when the researcher informs the subject of all aspects of a study and allows the subject to choose whether to participate and whether to withdraw from the study at any time without penalty
3. This right is violated if the subject is coerced into participating, becomes a subject without realizing it, or is deceived in any way about the research

C. Right to privacy
1. The right to privacy is an individual's freedom to determine when and how much private information will be shared
2. This right is protected when an informed subject voluntarily shares private information
3. This right is violated when private information is obtained without the subject's knowledge or against the subject's will

D. Right to anonymity or confidentiality
1. The researcher is responsible for keeping obtained information and the subject's identity private
2. Anonymity is maintained if the researcher does not know the subject's identity; confidentiality is ensured if the subject's name is separated from the data

SEARCHING THE WEB
More on federal guidelines

A summary of the National Research Act (Pub. L. 93-348) and The Belmont Report can be found at www.nih.gov/grants/oprr/belmont.htm.

3. This right is protected by analyzing data according to groups or reporting findings so that individual responses cannot be recognized
4. This right is violated when an unauthorized person gains access to personal information
5. Violations of this right may harm the subject and lead to loss of trust in the researcher or research study

E. Right to fair treatment
1. The researcher is responsible for selecting and treating all subjects in the same unbiased manner
2. To ensure fair treatment, the researcher must ensure that subjects know beforehand their expected roles and how the researcher plans to interact in the study
3. This right is protected by random selection of subjects
4. This right is violated when subjects are selected because they are easily manipulated or because of another reason unrelated to the study

F. Right to protection from harm
1. The researcher is responsible for protecting the subject from unnecessary discomfort or injury resulting from the study
2. This right is protected by the researcher's attempts to maximize a study's potential benefits and minimize its risks
3. This right is violated when the risks to subjects outweigh the benefits

◆ VI. Informed consent

A. General information
1. All researchers are required to obtain informed consent from all participating subjects
2. Informed consent (oral or written) implies that subjects have sufficient information, are able to comprehend the information, and have free choice to participate

B. Key elements of an informed consent
1. The study's purpose
2. The researcher's qualifications
3. The population being studied and the reasons for selecting it
4. A description of how and why the individual was selected for the study

5. An explanation of the procedures used
6. The time required for participation
7. The risks related to participation
8. The benefits that reasonably can be expected from participation
9. The alternative procedures, if any, that might benefit the subject
10. The procedure for maintaining anonymity or confidentiality
11. The availability of treatments should injury result
12. The person to contact for answers to questions, concerns about human rights, or follow-up treatment of injuries resulting from the research
13. The subject's freedom to choose whether to participate or withdraw

POINTS TO REMEMBER

♦ Unethical experiments and mistreatment of human research subjects influenced the development of professional guidelines and ethical codes.

♦ The American Nurses Association Human Rights Guidelines is the only professional code to identify the rights of subjects and nurses involved in research.

♦ Any organization that receives federal funding and performs research with human subjects must have an institutional review board to protect the subjects' rights.

♦ Each human subject has the right to self-determination, privacy, anonymity or confidentiality, fair treatment, and protection from harm.

♦ Children and persons who are terminally ill, mentally impaired, or institutionalized are considered vulnerable subjects and consequently require extra protection.

STUDY QUESTIONS

To evaluate your understanding of this chapter, answer the following questions in the space provided; compare your responses with the correct answers in appendix B, pages 237 to 244.

1. Which experimental studies are noted for their unethical treatment of human subjects? _____

_____

_____

2. What international code resulted from the unethical experimentation spotlighted during the Nazi criminal trials? _____

_____

_____

3. What three ethical principles are relevant to research? _____

_____

_____

4. What human rights require protection in ethical research? _____

_____

_____

CRITICAL THINKING AND APPLICATION EXERCISES

1. Read a research consent form. Does it contain all the key elements required for informed consent?

2. Read a research article. Consider the potential risks and benefits for the subjects who participated.

3. Discuss the ethical implications that should be considered if a large tobacco company funded a study on the effects of smoking on lung cancer.

4. Consider ways in which the following human rights might be violated:

   a. Right to self-determination

   b. Right to privacy

   c. Right to anonymity or confidentiality

   d. Right to fair treatment

   e. Right to protection from harm

5. Describe steps you might take to protect the human rights listed above.

15

Research Problem Selection

LEARNING OBJECTIVES

After studying this chapter, you should be able to:

♦ Identify how nurse researchers select and formulate research problems.

♦ Describe the information found in the problem of a study.

♦ List four sources for nursing research problems.

♦ Describe the factors to consider when selecting a research problem.

♦ List pertinent questions to ask when critiquing a research problem and purpose statement.

CHAPTER OVERVIEW

This chapter identifies the process used to select and formulate research problems. It lists several sources for research problems and outlines important factors to consider when selecting a research problem. Formulation of the purpose statement is described, and pertinent questions to consider when critiquing the problem and purpose statement of a research study are listed.

♦ I. Introduction

A. One of the most important steps in research is selecting the problem and formulating the purpose statement

1. The researcher selects a topic and narrows it into a specific problem

134

2. The problem identifies the area of concern and provides direction for the entire study
3. The problem guides the study toward a quantitative or qualitative approach
4. The problem must be stated clearly before it can be solved

B. The ability to wonder about situations helps the researcher identify research problems

C. After deciding *what* to study, the researcher begins formulating *why* to conduct the research

D. The problem of the study clarifies a number of issues
1. The extent of the problem
2. The significance of the problem
3. The rationale for the study
4. The researcher's intentions
5. The clinical context of the study
6. The ways in which findings will be used

E. The problem typically concludes with the purpose statement

♦ II. Sources for research problems

A. General information
1. To identify research problems, the researcher must be aware of personal thoughts, observations, and everyday experiences that signal potential areas of concern
2. Primary sources for research problems include nursing practice, literature, theory, and interactions with peers and researchers

B. Sources in nursing practice
1. Questions about patient care
2. Observations of patient and nurse behaviors
3. Patient care conferences
4. Complaints and expressions of dissatisfaction from patients and staff
5. Current nursing procedures compared with new techniques
6. Chart reviews

C. Literature sources
1. Journals and textbooks
2. Abstracts
3. THESES and DISSERTATIONS
4. Internet

D. Theory sources
1. The work of nursing theorists
2. Theories developed in other disciplines
3. Personal theories

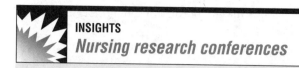

INSIGHTS

Nursing research conferences

Nursing research conferences may be an especially valuable source for identify-ing research problems. At these conferences, current research findings are reported, and they stimulate ideas for replication, extension, or related research problems.

E. Sources involving interactions with peers and researchers
   1. Formal educational experiences
   2. Professional workshops and presentations
   3. Staff-development education and orientation programs
   4. Policy and procedure committee meetings
   5. Journal clubs (see *Nursing research conferences*)

♦ **III. Selecting a research problem**

A. General information
   1. The selection of a research problem is not determined by specific rules
   2. The most important factors to consider are the problem's signifi-cance, researchability, feasibility, and interest to the researcher

B. Considerations related to significance
   1. Will conducting the study expand nursing's knowledge base?
   2. Will conducting the study improve nursing practice or policy?
   3. Will conducting the study benefit patients, nurses, or society?

C. Considerations related to researchability
   1. The problem should not involve ethical or moral issues
   2. All problems should be capable of being defined and measured
   3. The problem should be specific enough to be manageable

D. Considerations related to feasibility
   1. The study should be able to be completed within the allotted time
   2. Willing subjects should be available to participate in the study
   3. Sufficient funding, facilities, and equipment should be available
   4. The researcher should have the expertise required
   5. Coworkers should be available and willing to cooperate
   6. No unfair or unethical demands should be imposed

E. Considerations related to researcher's interest
   1. Levels of enthusiasm can be expected to rise and fall
   2. Unless the problem is especially interesting and appealing, the re-searcher may find the study too tedious or too difficult to complete

CHECKLIST
Problem and purpose statement

Use the following questions to critique the research problem and purpose statement of a study.

	Yes	No
• Does the researcher describe the problem's significance to nursing?	☐	☐
• Has the researcher outlined the rationale for conducting the study?	☐	☐
• Does the purpose statement clearly identify the population and the variables being studied?	☐	☐
• Does the purpose statement express a relationship between the variables?	☐	☐
• Does the purpose statement suggest empirical testability?	☐	☐
• Has the researcher considered practical issues, such as time, funding, facilities, equipment, and the cooperation of others?	☐	☐

◆ IV. Formulating the purpose statement

A. General information
   1. The researcher should write the research problem and purpose statement before beginning the study (see *Problem and purpose statement*)
   2. Writing the purpose statement may help the researcher to pinpoint uncertainties that need clarification before the study can proceed

B. Objectives of the purpose statement
   1. To provide direction to the research study
   2. To specify what the researcher will examine
   3. To help any user of the research evaluate the study

C. Items typically included in the purpose statement
   1. VARIABLES to be studied and their relationships
   2. Specifics about the population being studied
   3. The possibility of using EMPIRICAL TESTING

D. Forms of the purpose statement
   1. The *interrogative* form poses the purpose as a question
   2. The *declarative* form expresses the purpose as a statement

E. Correlational or comparative statements
   1. A *correlational* statement discusses the possibility of a relationship between the variables and may be predictive

SEARCHING THE WEB
Nursing research ideas

Use a search engine such as AltaVista, Excite, Hotbot, InfoSeek, Lycos, or Yahoo to surf the Web for nursing research ideas and to learn what research is being conducted around the world. A search engine checks each page or representative pages on every Web site and "reads" them, then creates an index from the pages that have been read. When the search engine receives your search request, it compares your request to the entries in the index and returns results to you.

2. A *comparative* purpose statement discusses the possibility of a difference between the variables and may be causal

F. The purpose statement for a qualitative study may simply identify the area of concern requiring study

POINTS TO REMEMBER

♦ Selecting a research problem is a key step in the research process.

♦ After the researcher has identified a problem to study, the problem is refined and narrowed to a specific topic.

♦ The introduction of the study should describe the problem and indicate why it is being researched.

♦ The problem should be significant, researchable, feasible, and interesting to the researcher.

♦ The purpose statement should identify the key variables, specify the population being studied, and imply whether empirical testing is possible.

STUDY QUESTIONS

To evaluate your understanding of this chapter, answer the following questions in the space provided; compare your responses with the correct answers in appendix B, pages 237 to 244.

1. Why is research problem identification an important step? _____

_____

_____

2. What are possible sources for a research problem? _____

_____

_____

3. Which factors should be considered when selecting a research problem? __

_____

_____

4. What two forms might a purpose statement take? _____

_____

_____

CRITICAL THINKING AND APPLICATION EXERCISES

1. Read the introduction to a research article. Use the checklist on page 137 to critique the problem and purpose statement.

2. Consider patient care that you have recently delivered. What questions do you have about the care that might be answered by a research study?

3. Review a nursing procedure and consider alternative methods that might be used in the procedure. Could a comparison of the methods be a problem for a research study?

4. Consider the significance, researchability, and feasibility for the research problem identified above.

5. Write a purpose statement for the research problem identified above.

16

Literature Review

LEARNING OBJECTIVES

After studying this chapter, you should be able to:

♦ Explain why a researcher conducts a literature review.

♦ Explain research findings, theoretical information, methodological information, opinion articles, and anecdotal descriptions.

♦ Describe methods for organizing the information and the mechanics of writing the review.

♦ Discuss initial and secondary searches.

♦ Explain how to conduct manual and computer literature searches.

♦ Identify criteria for critiquing a literature review.

CHAPTER OVERVIEW

This chapter outlines the principles related to reviewing research literature. Several purposes for conducting a review are discussed, and the processes involved in performing a literature review are described. Aspects of both manual and computer literature searches are included. Pertinent questions to consider when critiquing a literature review are listed.

♦ I. Introduction

A. In quantitative research, the LITERATURE REVIEW is done at the start and lays the foundation for the research project

B. In qualitative research, the literature review may be done during or after data are analyzed; the literature is compared and contrasted with the study findings (see chapters 19 and 22)

C. The researcher conducts the review by thoroughly examining all available scientific and theoretical information related to the research problem

1. The amount of available literature depends on how well the topic has been researched previously

2. A short, well-organized review of pertinent studies is more valuable than a long, rambling review of irrelevant studies

D. A thorough review should include primary and secondary sources

1. PRIMARY SOURCES, containing original research findings, are preferred and should be used whenever possible

2. SECONDARY SOURCES, containing interpretations of research findings, are helpful in providing bibliographic information

♦ II. Purposes of the review

A. General information

1. The primary purpose of a literature review is to help the researcher gauge what is known and unknown about the research problem

2. A review can serve many additional purposes

a. Help the researcher to identify or refine the research problem

b. Strengthen the rationale for the research

c. Develop a framework for the study

d. Provide a useful approach to conducting the study

e. Explain or support the findings

B. Identifying or refining the research problem

1. Reading clinically related literature may help the researcher to recognize areas that need further research and study

2. The research problem may be refined during the literature review

C. Strengthening the rationale for the research

1. A lack of literature related to the problem may indicate that the problem needs further study

2. Conversely, the researcher may find that the problem has been extensively researched, indicating that another study is unnecessary

D. Developing a framework for the study

1. In reviewing the literature, the researcher may discover a theory to serve as an approach to the study

2. The review may lead the researcher to formulate ideas about how the research problem and concepts are linked

E. Providing a useful approach to conducting the study

1. The literature review may reveal specific research strategies and procedures used in previous studies

2. The researcher may be able to adapt an approach used in a previous study or develop a new approach to conducting the research

F. Explaining or supporting the findings

1. The literature review may reveal findings that are similar to or different from those obtained in the current study

2. The literature review may be used to verify relationships and theories that emerged from the data obtained in the study

♦ III. Review process

A. General information

1. The researcher conducts a search or a series of searches to find relevant references

2. The researcher should pursue as many relevant references as possible when conducting a literature review

3. The researcher reviews all the available information and decides which references to include in the written review

B. Types of information to review

1. Research findings from previous related studies

2. Theoretical information concerning broader problem issues

3. Methodological information on research methods previously used

4. Opinion articles discussing specific viewpoints or attitudes about the problem; the researcher should keep in mind their subjectivity and limited use

5. Anecdotal descriptions of others' experiences; the researcher should keep in mind their limited use

C. Conducting an initial search

1. In an initial search, the researcher scans pertinent publications, including indexes to nursing and health care literature, bibliographies, ABSTRACTS, and other primary and secondary sources, to develop an overview of knowledge available on the problem

2. The initial review also helps the researcher to determine whether the problem has already been thoroughly studied, whether necessary instruments and tools are available to measure the variables, and whether ideas and beliefs about the problem are correct

3. This step enables the researcher to decide whether to proceed with the study

D. Conducting a secondary search

1. In a secondary search, the researcher makes a concerted effort to review all published information related to the problem

SEARCHING THE WEB
Nursing and allied health literature

membership fee, CINAHL has direct on-line service. The CINAHL
ation Systems can be found at http://cinahl.com.

. *Dissertation Abstracts Online* corresponds with the information found
in *Dissertation Abstracts International* from 1861 to the present
. *CATLINE* contains references for books and serials cataloged at the
National Library of Medicine
. *BIOETHICSLINE* includes citations from 1973 to the present concerning ethical questions in health care housed at the National Library of Medicine and the Kennedy Institute of Ethics
. Several additional databases are available for searching selected areas
in health and sciences

'irginia Henderson International Nursing Library
. Sigma Theta Tau established the library to be a computerized collection of databases and knowledge resources
. The library contains an on-line network and electronic journal
. The electronic databases include Directory of Nurse Researchers,
Research Conference Proceedings, Sigma Theta Tau International
Grant Recipients and Projects, Information Resources Database,
and tables of contents of *IMAGE: Journal of Nursing Scholarship*
. Subscribers can also access other services, such as Online Conferencing, and read the Sigma Theta Tau International News

nternet
. The Internet has varying levels of usefulness for researchers
. Accessing the World Wide Web requires a modem, basic communications software, and a commercial on-line service, called an Internet service provider
. Some Internet services may require additional software or subscription fees

POINTS TO REMEMBER

ature review demonstrates what is known about a research problem
lidates the need for the current study.

ypes of information reviewed include research findings, theoretical in-
tion, methodological information, opinion articles, and anecdotal de-
ons.

2. The researcher typically begins by searching for the most recent
publications

E. Evaluating the information
1. All references should be summarized and classified for easy retrieval
2. Reading the abstract or summary is a reliable way to determine the
potential usefulness of an article
3. The reviewer's notes, typically made on index cards or typed into a
computer, should include a synopsis of each article along with all bibliographic information and should be organized according to categories

F. Writing a literature review
1. Before writing the review, the researcher selects appropriate sources
from related literature
a. The researcher typically selects sources based on their relevance to
the problem and the study's purpose statement
b. The researcher typically organizes the selected sources according
to variable, theoretical or research classification, ability to support
the study's framework, or ability to explain the study's finding
2. The researcher typically develops an outline as a guide for writing
the introduction, body, and summary of the literature review
3. The introduction describes the organization and purpose of the review
4. The body, which contains a detailed analysis of relevant studies, typically focuses on research and theoretical information
5. In the body, the researcher compares and contrasts studies with similar methodology or results, pointing out consistencies and contradictions while striving for objectivity; the researcher should try to
present the studies logically, remembering to relate each study to
others and to paraphrase material whenever possible
6. The summary typically discusses the quality of the literature reviewed, identifies gaps in knowledge, and demonstrates the need for
the study (see *Literature Review,* page 144, and *Securing nursing research,* page 145)

◆ IV. Manual literature search

A. General information
1. A manual search, which is typically time-consuming but relatively
inexpensive, is a hands-on way to locate and review literature
2. This type of search requires familiarity with the library and various
index tools, such as card catalogs, medical and nursing indexes, abstracts, and bibliographies

B. Card catalogs
1. A card catalog is the main source for locating resources in a library
2. In most libraries, the card catalog is listed on an online computer

CHECKLIST
Literature review

Use the following questions to critique the literature review portion of a study.

	Yes	No
• Does the literature review immediately follow the introduction and purpose statement?	☐	☐
• Are all the major variables included in the review?	☐	☐
• Did the researcher use mostly primary sources?	☐	☐
• Did the review include recent literature?	☐	☐
• Did the researcher include most major studies conducted on the problem?	☐	☐
• Did the researcher include mostly theoretical or research articles rather than opinion or anecdotal articles?	☐	☐
• Did the researcher include a summary that critically evaluates the literature, identifies gaps, and demonstrates how the current study will fill the gaps?	☐	☐
• Is the review logically organized and objective?	☐	☐

C. Indexes
  1. Indexes are usually organized according to subject and author
  2. Indexes are the main source for locating articles published in journals
  3. A number of indexes are of key importance to nursing researchers
     a. *Cumulative Index to Nursing and Allied Health Literature* includes listings from more than 300 nursing and allied health journals
     b. *International Nursing Index* includes listings on nursing literature from around the world
     c. *Nursing Studies Index* includes listings on nursing literature from 1900 to 1959
     d. *Index Medicus* includes more than 3,000 biomedical journals
     e. *Hospital and Health Administration Index* contains references on health care planning, administration, and delivery of care

D. Abstracts (brief synopses of articles)
  1. *Nursing Research Abstracts,* published from 1960 to 1978, in *Nursing Research* journal, contains abstracts of nursing-related studies
  2. *Nursing Abstracts* contains abstracts of significant nursing research studies published since 1979

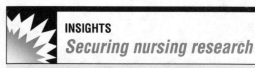

INSIGHTS
Securing nursing research

For nursing science to be cumulative, synthesis of the exis̸
is essential. Sound reviewing strategies must be valued an̸
Conflicting findings should be explored, quantitative and q̸
be included, and conceptual clarity maintained.

  3. *Psychological Abstracts* includes abstracts from̸
     lications in psychology and related disciplines̸
  4. *Dissertation Abstracts International* includes al̸
     dissertations published throughout the world̸

E. Bibliographies
  1. Bibliographies contain lists of publications o̸
  2. They are included in bibliographic indexes as̸
     most research articles, books, theses, and diss̸

♦ **V. Computer literature search**

A. General information
  1. Computer searches are used to access bibliog̸
     has been stored in DATABASES
  2. A computer search can be done at any library̸
     database; a microcomputer equipped with a̸
     cations software also may be used to search n̸
  3. To locate appropriate information, the resear̸
     topic and determine key words to use in the̸
  4. Cost depends on the database searched and t̸
  5. Advanced technology has made computer se̸
     comprehensive, and invaluable

B. Databases
  1. *CINAHL (Nursing & Allied Health)* correspo̸
     tion found in *Cumulative Index to Nursing a̸
     ture* from 1982 to the present
  2. *MEDLINE* corresponds with the informatio̸
     Medicus, International Nursing Index, and *In̸
     from 1966 to the present
  3. *AIDSLINE* covers AIDS literature on-line̸
  4. *HealthSTAR* (merged: AHA, Health Plannin̸
     [HEALTH], and Health Service/Technolog̸
     [HSTAR])
  5. *ERIC* corresponds with the information fou̸
     cation and *Research in Education* from 1966̸

♦ Notes should be systematically recorded and categorized for easy retrieval of information.

♦ The written literature review should be logically organized and objective and should contain mostly research and theoretical sources.

♦ Sources may be searched manually in card catalogs, indexes, abstracts, and bibliographies or by computer through databases.

STUDY QUESTIONS

To evaluate your understanding of this chapter, answer the following questions in the space provided; compare your responses with the correct answers in appendix B, pages 237 to 244.

1. Why does a researcher conduct a literature review? _____
   _____
   _____

2. What purposes might a literature review serve? _____
   _____
   _____

3. What types of literature might the researcher review? _____
   _____
   _____

4. What are the advantages of a computer search over a manual search?
   _____
   _____

CRITICAL THINKING AND APPLICATION EXERCISES

1. Examine the reference list in a research article. Determine which citations are primary sources and which are secondary sources. What criteria did you use to make your decision?

2. Retrieve at least six research articles identified on the above search. Write a two- to three-paragraph review synthesizing the findings from the studies.

3. Read the literature review from a research article. Use the checklist on page 144 to critique the review.

17

Conceptual and Theoretical Frameworks

CHAPTER OVERVIEW

This chapter describes the use of conceptual and theoretical frameworks in nursing research and explains the four key concepts of particular interest to nursing. It outlines the purposes and uses of conceptual and theoretical frameworks, and discusses nursing and adapted frameworks. Examples are provided as well. Problems related to frameworks are presented, and pertinent questions to consider when critiquing frameworks are listed.

♦ I. Introduction

A. A framework, also called a frame of reference, is the logical but abstract structure of a research study

1. In quantitative research, the framework is a testable theory
2. In qualitative research, the framework is a philosophy, and a theory may be developed as an outcome of the study

B. The framework helps the researcher to organize the study and interpret the results

1. The researcher uses the framework as a guide through the entire research process, beginning with the HYPOTHESIS or research question and ending with the study's conclusions
2. The researcher organizes and explains all of the information acquired in the study through the framework's context
3. Working within a framework enables the researcher to link the research to nursing's body of knowledge, allowing the findings to have meaning beyond the specific study (see *The relationship of theory and research,* page 150)

C. All frameworks are based on the identification of key CONCEPTS and the relationships between or among those concepts

1. Concepts typically are abstract (such as "pain" or "grief"), but they can also be concrete (such as "temperature" or "weight")
2. The researcher formulates PROPOSITIONS to identify relationships between concepts

D. Four key concepts — person, environment, health, and nursing — are of particular interest to nursing researchers

1. *Person,* the recipient of nursing care, may be an individual, a family, or a community
2. *Environment,* the setting in which nursing occurs, typically revolves around the person's significant others and surroundings
3. *Health,* the person's state of wellness or illness, is identified as the purpose of nursing
4. *Nursing,* the actions taken by nurses to benefit the person

E. A framework can derive from related concepts (conceptual) or an existing THEORY (theoretical)

1. Although the terms conceptual framework and theoretical framework are sometimes used interchangeably, they have different meanings
2. CONCEPTUAL FRAMEWORKS, usually less formal than theoretical frameworks, are used for studies in which existing theory is inapplicable or insufficient
3. *Theoretical frameworks,* usually more formal than conceptual frameworks, are used for studies based on existing theories
4. Conceptual and theoretical frameworks may be represented as models

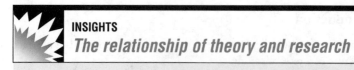

INSIGHTS
The relationship of theory and research

In *The Relationship of Theory and Research* (1986), Fawcett and Downs state that a close connection between theory and research exists. The purpose of research is to test or generate theory. Research relies on theory, and the development of theory depends on research. Research is the method for gathering data required for a theory. Theory without research and research without theory do little to advance nursing's knowledge base.

    a. A MODEL is a symbolic representation that helps to express abstract concepts and relationships easily, using minimal words
    b. A model can be represented schematically (using boxes, arrows, or other symbols) or statistically (using letters, numbers, and mathematical symbols)

♦ II. Conceptual frameworks

A. General information
    1. A conceptual framework may be derived from empirical observation, intuition, or literature
    2. The researcher develops the framework by identifying and clarifying the concepts to be used in the study, then specifying the proposed relationships among the concepts
    3. A conceptual framework may be more global and abstract than a theoretical framework

B. Purposes of conceptual frameworks
    1. To clarify concepts and propose relationships among the concepts
    2. To provide a context for interpreting the study findings
    3. To explain observations
    4. To encourage theory development

C. Uses of conceptual frameworks in nursing
    1. Expanding nursing's knowledge base
    2. Defining nursing
    3. Providing a framework when existing theory is insufficient
    4. Clarifying concepts and the relationships among those concepts
    5. Helping nurses provide patient care

♦ III. Theoretical frameworks

A. General information
    1. A theoretical framework is based on a theory derived from specific concepts and propositions that are induced or deduced

    2. Theories are always invented, never discovered; they can be tested but never proved

B. Purposes of theoretical frameworks
    1. To test theories
    2. To make research findings meaningful beyond the present study
    3. To explain observations
    4. To predict and control situations
    5. To stimulate research and expand nursing's knowledge base

C. Uses of theoretical frameworks in nursing
    1. Expanding nursing's knowledge base
    2. Defining nursing
    3. Clarifying concepts
    4. Formulating hypotheses for testing
    5. Helping nurses provide patient care

♦ IV. Conceptual and theoretical frameworks used in nursing research

A. General information
    1. Nursing researchers use conceptual and theoretical frameworks developed by nurses and other professionals
    2. Nursing frameworks create formal explanations of what constitutes the profession of nursing
        a. Nursing frameworks vary in the way they define and link key concepts and in the way they emphasize some relationships over others
        b. Nursing frameworks are relatively recent and are still being developed
        c. Researchers need to test nursing frameworks to help formulate and refine nursing theories, making them more useful to nursing practice
    3. Nursing researchers may use frameworks from other disciplines that can be adapted to nursing-related concepts
        a. These disciplines include psychology, sociology, education, physiology, and anthropology
        b. Adapted frameworks are sometimes referred to as borrowed or shared

B. Examples of nursing frameworks
    1. M. Rogers' "Science of Unitary Human Beings"
    2. D. Orem's "Self-Care Model"
    3. C. Roy's "Adaptation Model"
    4. I. King's "Theory of Goal Attainment"
    5. D. Johnson's "Behavioral Systems Model"
    6. M. Levine's "Conservation Theory"

SEARCHING THE WEB
Nursing theories and theorists

If you want to discuss a particular theory or nurse theorist, search your on-line service for a chat room, or start your own chat room where you can talk with colleagues about the theory that interests you.

7. B. Neuman's "Health Care Systems Model"
8. H. Peplau's "Interpersonal Relations in Nursing"
9. J. Paterson's and L. Zderad's "Humanistic Nursing Theory"
10. M. Leininger's "Culture Care Diversity and Universality"
11 J. Watson's "Philosophy of Science and Caring"
12. R. Parse's "Human Becoming Theory"
13. M. Newman's "Health as Expanding Consciousness"
14. N. Pender's "Health Promotion Model"

C. Examples of adapted frameworks
1. A. Bandura's "Social Learning Theory"
2. A. Maslow's "Hierarchy of Human Needs"
3. L. Festinger's "Cognitive Dissonance"
4. M. Seligman's "Helplessness"
5. E. Duvall's and S. Minuchin's family theories
6. V. Satir's "Family Communication Theory"
7. R. Melzack's and D. Wall's "Pain"
8. J. Piaget's, S. Freud's, and E. Erikson's developmental theories
9. C. Spielberger's "Anxiety"
10. I. Rosenstock's and M. Becker's "Health Beliefs and Compliance"
11. R. Lazarus' and H. Selye's stress theories

◆ V. Problems related to conceptual and theoretical frameworks

A. General information
1. Framework problems typically result from researcher inexperience
2. Such problems may limit the study's usefulness because the findings may have no significance beyond the scope of the individual study
3. Common problems include use of an inappropriate or unidentified framework in a study, use of a framework that is disconnected from the study, and use of multiple frameworks within the same study

B. Use of an inappropriate framework
1. Typically occurs when the researcher tries to make a research problem fit within the context of a framework that may be only marginally related to the study

CHECKLIST

Conceptual and theoretical frameworks

Use the following questions to critique the conceptual or theoretical framework used in a study.

	Yes	No
• Is the framework clearly identified?	☐	☐
• Are the concepts and propositions clearly outlined?	☐	☐
• Does the framework appear to be appropriate for the research problem?	☐	☐
• Is sufficient literature presented to support and justify the framework?	☐	☐
• Did the researcher use a nursing framework or a borrowed framework?	☐	☐
• Does the link between the problem and the framework seem plausible and uncontrived?	☐	☐
• Does the hypothesis or research question flow naturally from the framework?	☐	☐
• Was the framework used to guide the research design, data collection and analysis, and interpretation of the findings?	☐	☐
• If the study findings do not support the framework, does the researcher suggest plausible explanations for this discrepancy?	☐	☐

    2. Framework may be useless in interpreting the study's results

C. Use of a disconnected framework
    1. Typically occurs when the researcher fails to connect an appropriately developed framework with the study
    2. Framework has no meaning in the study and consequently is useless

D. Use of an unidentified framework
    1. Typically occurs when the researcher fails to outline a framework
    2. Results in findings that have no basis for generalizing to other situations

E. Use of multiple frameworks
    1. Typically occurs when the researcher tries to use two or more frameworks for the same study
    2. Framework has no meaning within the study because of the lack of logical connections between or among the frameworks (see *Conceptual and theoretical frameworks*)

POINTS TO REMEMBER

♦ A framework gives direction to a study, provides a context for interpreting the findings, and adds to nursing's knowledge base.

♦ Person, environment, health, and nursing—four key concepts of interest to nursing—are the focus of many frameworks used in research studies.

♦ The main purpose of a conceptual or theoretical framework is to make research findings meaningful beyond the present study.

♦ A theoretical framework is more specific and concrete than a conceptual framework.

♦ A model is a symbolic representation of a framework.

♦ Use of an inappropriate or unidentified framework, a disconnected framework, or multiple frameworks within a study may compromise the study's usefulness.

STUDY QUESTIONS

To evaluate your understanding of this chapter, answer the following questions in the space provided; compare your responses with the correct answers in appendix B, pages 237 to 244.

1. Which key concepts are of particular interest to nursing researchers?_____

_____

_____

2. What is the difference between a schematic model and a mathematical model? _____

_____

_____

3. What is the difference between the base for conceptual frameworks and the base for theoretical frameworks? _____

_____

_____

4. What are four nursing theories used to guide nursing research?

_____

_____

5. What are four theories borrowed from other disciplines used to guide nursing research?_____

_____

_____

6. What common problems are related to conceptual and theoretical frameworks?_____

_____

_____

CRITICAL THINKING AND APPLICATION EXERCISES

1. Review one example of a nursing framework. Determine how the key concepts — person, environment, health, and nursing — are defined.

2. Review one example of a nursing framework. Consider how it could be used to guide a research study.

3. Review one of the examples of an adapted framework. Consider how it could be used to guide a nursing research study.

4. Read the framework from a research article. Draw a model to represent the concepts and relationships.

5. Read the framework from a quantitative research article. Use the checklist on page 153 to critique the framework.

18

Variables, Hypotheses, and Research Questions

CHAPTER OVERVIEW

This chapter considers the relationships among variables, hypotheses, and research questions. It also details six types of variables and defines the difference between theoretical and operational definitions. Six types of hypotheses are described, and simple examples are provided. The role of research questions is discussed, and hypotheses are compared with research questions. Pertinent questions to consider when critiquing hypotheses and research questions are listed.

♦ I. Introduction

A. QUANTITATIVE RESEARCH is based on the examination of relationships between the specific variables identified in a study

    1. A *variable* is a concept examined in a particular research study (for example, sex, age, heart rate, or pain perception)

    2. All variables must be concretely defined before they can be studied and measured

    3. Variables in qualitative studies may be abstract

B. The researcher hypothesizes about the relationships between variables before beginning the study

    1. A *hypothesis* is a statement that predicts a relationship among two or more variables identified in the purpose statement

    2. The hypothesis is more concise than the purpose statement

C. Research questions may be used instead of hypotheses whenever the researcher has insufficient knowledge to formulate a hypothesis; they are frequently used in qualitative research (see *Hypotheses and research questions,* page 158)

♦ II. Research variables

A. General information

    1. All variables may be quantified and converted mathematically for statistical analysis

    2. All variables must be defined theoretically and operationally to reduce bias and clearly communicate meaning

    3. THEORETICAL DEFINITIONS, which are broad and abstract, derive from a specific theory or nursing-related literature; for example, "anxiety" may be defined theoretically as "a feeling of uneasiness or apprehension that affects body processes"

    4. OPERATIONAL DEFINITIONS reflect the procedures or acts that the researcher performs to measure the existence or degree of a variable; for example, "anxiety" may be defined operationally as "a state of mind that causes systolic blood pressure to increase at least 10 points"

B. Types of variables

    1. An *independent* variable is the presumed cause or influencing factor; it is manipulated by the researcher in experimental research

    2. A *dependent* variable is the response or outcome the researcher wishes to explain or predict

    3. A *continuous* variable can take on a range of different values that can be represented on a continuum

CHECKLIST
Hypotheses and research questions

Use the following questions to critique the hypotheses and research questions found in a study.

	Yes	No
• Does the research report contain hypotheses or research questions?	☐	☐
• Do the hypotheses or research questions flow from the conceptual or theoretical framework or the literature review?	☐	☐
• Do the hypotheses predict solutions to the problem?	☐	☐
• Are the hypotheses clearly and objectively stated in a declarative form?	☐	☐
• Are the variables identified and potentially measurable?	☐	☐
• Do the hypotheses predict a relationship between the variables?	☐	☐
• Do the hypotheses indicate the population being studied?	☐	☐
• Are the hypotheses testable and clearly supported?	☐	☐
• If the hypotheses are nondirectional, did the researcher present a rationale to support their use?	☐	☐
• Are the hypotheses stated in the research form rather than the null form?	☐	☐
• Are the independent and dependent variables theoretically and operationally defined?	☐	☐
• Are the definitions consistent with the theoretical framework and the literature?	☐	☐

4. A *categorical* variable has a limited range of values that are represented by discrete categories

5. An *extraneous* variable is a factor that can affect the dependent variable and interfere with the results

6. A *confounding* variable is an extraneous factor that has not been controlled

♦ III. Hypotheses

A. General information

1. Hypotheses, formal statements of the expected relationships between the variables, provide direction for gathering and interpreting data; they are derived through inductive or deductive reasoning

2. The researcher should write the hypothesis before collecting the data and never alter the hypothesis after analyzing the data

3. The researcher should formulate as many hypotheses as needed to address all aspects of the research problem; the number of hypotheses formulated usually reflects the researcher's expertise and the complexity of the research problem

B. Purposes of hypotheses

1. Help direct the research study by the following

a. Identifying the population and specifying the variables

b. Guiding the research design selection

c. Suggesting an appropriate sampling technique and data collection and analysis methods

d. Guiding the interpretation of results

2. Help link theory to reality and, once confirmed, lend support to a theory

C. Sources of hypotheses

1. Conceptual or theoretical frameworks, the most important sources, enable the researcher to derive hypotheses from concepts or theories

2. Personal experience enables the researcher to induce hypotheses by observing events and explaining or predicting the relationship between events

3. The literature review enables the researcher to formulate new hypotheses by regenerating hypotheses from other related studies or testing the assumptions underlying such studies

D. Characteristics of a hypothesis

1. Written as a declarative sentence, commonly using a present-tense verb; content should be similar to that of the purpose statement

2. Identifies the population to be studied

3. Identifies at least one independent variable and one dependent variable

4. Is empirically testable and therefore cannot focus on moral or ethical issues

E. Types of hypotheses

1. *Simple* hypothesis

a. Easy to analyze

b. Predicts a relationship between one independent variable and one dependent variable (for example, "a" is caused by "b")

2. *Complex* hypothesis

a. Predicts the relationships among two or more independent variables and two or more dependent variables (for example, "a" and "b" are influenced by "c" and "d")

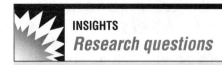

INSIGHTS
Research questions

The research question can help determine whether to use a quantitative or qualitative design. Questions addressing the exploration of a lived human experience would be answered using a qualitative design; those questions addressing differences between variables would be answered using a quantitative design.

     b. Often used in nursing research because it typically examines complex human situations and requires the identification of several variables

3. *Directional* hypothesis

     a. Can be simple or complex; predicts the direction of the relationship between the variables (for example, "a" is greater than "b")

     b. Form of most hypotheses deduced from theory

4. *Nondirectional* hypothesis

     a. Can be simple or complex; states that a relationship exists between the variables (for example, "a" is related to "b")

     b. Typically used when not enough is known about the problem to predict the direction of a relationship

5. *Research,* scientific, alternative, or theoretical hypothesis

     a. Can be simple or complex; usually is directional

     b. Anticipates a relationship between the variables

     c. Common form of hypotheses because of clarity

6. *Null* or statistical hypothesis

     a. Predicts that no relationship exists between the independent and dependent variables

     b. Used whenever statistical principles are used to draw conclusions

♦ IV. Research questions

A. General information

     1. The researcher may use a research question when knowledge is insufficient to formulate a hypothesis

     2. Research questions are commonly used in EXPLORATORY, DESCRIPTIVE, and qualitative research

     3. Questions guiding qualitative research are usually broad and abstract (see *Research questions*)

B. Characteristics of a research question

     1. Written as an interrogative sentence, using a present-tense verb

     2. Identifies the population

     3. Contains one or more variables

     4. Reflects the purpose statement

5. May or may not be empirically testable

6. Focuses on the variables and their possible relationships

♦ The researcher must be able to define the variables theoretically and operationally to test the hypothesis.

♦ The hypothesis predicts relationships among two or more variables and identifies the population to be studied.

♦ The hypothesis directs the research study and unifies theory and reality.

♦ Hypotheses are never proven; they are accepted or rejected, or supported or not supported.

♦ Hypotheses can be classified as simple, complex, directional, nondirectional, research, or null.

♦ Research questions may be used in exploratory, descriptive, or qualitative research or when insufficient knowledge is available to formulate hypotheses.

STUDY QUESTIONS

To evaluate your understanding of this chapter, answer the following questions in the space provided; compare your responses with the correct answers in appendix B, pages 237 to 244.

1. What is the relationship between a variable and a hypothesis? _____

_____

_____

2. What is the difference between the theoretical and operational definitions of a variable? _____

_____

_____

3. What is the difference between independent and dependent variables?

_____

_____

4. Why would a researcher use a complex hypothesis?_____

_____

_____

5. How might research questions used to guide qualitative studies differ from those used in quantitative research? _____

_____

_____

CRITICAL THINKING AND APPLICATION EXERCISES

1. Using back massage as an independent variable and pain as a dependent variable, write a hypothesis. Does it contain all of the characteristics outlined in section III. D?

2. Determine whether the hypothesis written above is simple or complex, directional or nondirectional, research or null.

3. Considering the variable pain, write a theoretical definition and an operational definition.

4. Read the research question from a qualitative research article. Use the checklist on page 158 to critique the research question.

5. Read the hypothesis from a quantitative research article. Use the checklist on page 158 to critique the hypothesis.

19

Research Designs

CHAPTER OVERVIEW

This chapter provides an overview of the various types of research designs. It presents threats to internal and external validity, and describes techniques used to control the threats. True experimental, quasi-experimental, pre-experimental, and nonexperimental quantitative research designs are outlined. Phenomenologic, grounded theory, ethnographic, historical, philosophical inquiry, and critical social theory qualitative research designs are presented. A discussion of other research designs includes cross-sectional, longitudinal, retrospective, prospective, survey, methodological, case study, secondary analysis, meta-analysis, and evaluation. Pertinent questions to consider when critiquing the various types of research designs are listed.

♦ I. Introduction

A. A research design is the logical plan used by the researcher to address the purpose statement in a research study

1. It follows an organized progression and takes the researcher from the research idea to the final step of the study
2. It determines specific strategies for obtaining subjects, collecting data, analyzing data, and interpreting results

B. Choosing a research design is a major research decision

C. All research designs address six basic elements

1. The setting in which the research occurs
2. The subjects to include in the research
3. The sample size or number of subjects in the study
4. The conditions under which data are collected
5. The methods used to collect the data
6. The researcher's plan for analyzing the findings

D. Most research designs are categorized as either quantitative or qualitative

1. *Quantitative* research, which is based on REDUCTIONISM, uses variables that are analyzed as numbers
2. *Qualitative* research, which is based on HOLISM, uses concepts that are analyzed as words to explore lived experiences
3. Many researchers think that qualitative research is more consistent with nursing's philosophical basis; others think that quantitative research is more rigorous and scientific
4. Quantitative research designs usually are best suited to studies that focus on determining relationships among variables; qualitative research designs, to studies that focus on discovery or exploration
5. Some researchers advocate integrating quantitative and qualitative research within a study or group of studies to enhance the knowledge gained

E. The researcher may also use triangulation

1. *Triangulation* is a strategy in which multiple methods are used in the research design to study the phenomenon and converge on the truth
2. There are five types of triangulation
   a. In *data triangulation,* data from several sources in a study are examined

INSIGHTS
Using designs to build a knowledge base

Researchers may use several designs to build a knowledge base in an area. For example, Fawcett used a qualitative design to begin a program of research to determine the needs of cesarean birth parents. Based on the initial findings, an antenatal education program was developed, tested, and refined using a variety of groups and settings. Finally, a quasi-experimental study was conducted to test the intervention.

b. In *investigator triangulation,* several investigators with differing backgrounds examine the same variables
c. In *theoretical triangulation,* several frameworks or perspectives are used in a study
d. In *methodological triangulation,* several methods, such as observations, interviews, and questionnaires, are used to collect data from the same subjects in a study
e. In *analysis triangulation,* different techniques are used to analyze the same data (see *Using designs to build a knowledge base*)

♦ II. Quantitative research designs

A. General information
1. The quantitative research design evolves from the hypothesis or research question and determines which methods and procedures will be used to select subjects, collect and analyze data, and interpret results
2. The main purposes are to help the researcher expand the knowledge base or find a solution to the research problem and maintain as much control as possible over all variables
3. Quantitative designs differ according to the degree of control the researcher has over the variables; the degree of control directly affects the internal and external validity of the study—two areas that help to determine whether the study results are credible and dependable
   a. *Internal validity,* the extent to which the effects detected in the study are a reflection of reality, depends on whether the effects on the dependent variable can be attributed to changes in the independent variable
   b. *External validity,* the extent to which the findings can be generalized beyond the sample used in the study, depends on whether the relationship between the independent and dependent variables can be applied to other populations or situations
   c. Factors other than the independent variable that affect the study results are referred to as *threats*
   (1) Threats to internal validity

        (a) History
        (b) Maturation
        (c) Testing
        (d) Instrumentation
        (e) Mortality or attrition
        (f) Selection bias
      (2) Threats to external validity
        (a) Sample inadequacy
        (b) Environmental influence

    4. Techniques used to control threats include the following

      a. *Randomization* is the random assignment of subjects to a group, with each individual in the population having an equal chance to be selected for the group

      b. *Homogeneity* is the selection for participation in a study of only those subjects who share an extraneous variable — for example, only men or only adults over age 65

      c. *Blocking* is the purposeful addition of an extraneous variable to the study's design — for example, random assignment of men and women to separate groups

      d. *Matching* is the formation of a comparison group by matching subjects on the basis of important extraneous variables — for example, age, sex, and health status

      e. *Analysis of covariance* is the control of extraneous variables through statistical procedures

    5. Quantitative research designs can be classified as true experimental, quasi-experimental, pre-experimental, and nonexperimental

B. True experimental designs

    1. A *true experimental design,* which offers the greatest amount of control and minimal threat to internal validity, allows the researcher to become actively involved in the study

    2. Characteristics of a true experimental design include the following

      a. *Manipulation* — the researcher manipulates the independent variable so that some of the subjects are affected

      b. *Control* — the researcher uses one or more measures to control the experiment, including the use of an unmanipulated control group that is compared with an experimental group

      c. *Randomization* — the researcher assigns subjects to groups by chance

    3. True experimental designs are the most effective method of testing cause-and-effect relationships

    4. *Causality* is based on meeting three criteria

      a. The cause must precede the effect

      b. An empirical relationship between the presumed cause and effect must exist

  c. The relationship cannot be attributable to the effect of a third
   variable
 5. True experimental designs can be classified into three types
  a. In a *pretest-posttest control group design,* the researcher randomly
   assigns each subject to either a control group or an experimental
   group
   (1) Both groups are given a pretest, after which only the experi-
    mental group receives a specific intervention that is manipu-
    lated by the researcher
   (2) Both groups are then given a posttest
   (3) The researcher examines the performances of both groups
    for changes in scores that may have resulted from the inter-
    vention
  b. In a *posttest-only control group design,* the researcher randomly assigns each subject to either a control group or an experimental
   group
   (1) After the experimental group receives a specific intervention,
    both groups are given a posttest
   (2) The researcher then examines the performances of both
    groups for differences in scores that may have resulted from
    the intervention
  c. In a *Solomon four-group design,* the researcher randomly assigns
   each subject to one of two control groups or one of two experimental groups
   (1) Only one control group or one experimental group is given
    the pretest, and both experimental groups receive a specific
    intervention
   (2) All groups are given a posttest
   (3) The researcher examines the performances of all the groups
    for the effect of the pretest on posttest scores and for any
    other differences among the groups
 6. Use of true experimental designs is limiting for a number of reasons
  a. Certain variables (such as age, sex, and height) cannot be physi-
   cally manipulated
  b. Other variables (such as disease or unhealthy habits) cannot be
   ethically manipulated
  c. True experimentation may be impossible in particular settings
  d. The HAWTHORNE EFFECT may interfere with the study's outcome
  e. Some researchers consider true experiments artificial and reduc-
   tionistic

C. Quasi-experimental designs
 1. A *quasi-experimental design* is used to test cause-and-effect relationships when true experimentation is impossible
  a. It is more conducive to a natural setting

    b. It allows the researcher to become actively involved in the study and to generalize the findings to an extent

2. Unlike a true experimental design, a quasi-experimental design does not depend on randomization or a control group; however, it does allow for manipulation of the independent variable and enables the researcher to introduce other factors to compensate for the lack of randomization or a control group

3. Typically, the researcher uses a comparison group instead of a control group to evaluate outcome differences

4. Quasi-experimental designs can be classified into two types

    a. A *nonequivalent control group design* is identical to the pretest-posttest control group of a true experimental design except that the subjects are not randomly assigned to groups

      (1) The researcher cannot assume that both groups are equal

      (2) The researcher therefore must rely on the results of a pretest to determine if groups are initially similar with respect to the dependent variable

    b. A *time series design* involves the collection of information from one group of subjects at several points over an extended period

      (1) The researcher introduces an intervention at a specific time during the course of data collection and evaluates the results based on information collected before and after the intervention

      (2) Although subjects are not randomly assigned, this design allows the researcher to manipulate factors to control the study

5. Use of quasi-experimental designs is limiting for two reasons

    a. The researcher cannot draw inferences about cause-and-effect relationships to the same degree as in true experimental designs

    b. The researcher has limited control over variables, which may necessitate formulating alternative explanations for the effect detected in the study

D. Pre-experimental designs

1. A *pre-experimental design*, which may be used when a control group is impossible or when limited opportunities for data collection are available, is typically more economical than a true experimental design or a quasi-experimental design

2. Pre-experimental designs can be classified according to two types

    a. A *posttest-only nonequivalent control group design* is similar to a nonequivalent control group quasi-experimental design except that the researcher has no pretest data with which to compare the groups' relationship to the dependent variable and has no basis on which to judge the initial equivalence or similarity of the two groups involved in the study

b. A *one-group pretest-posttest design* does not depend on the use of randomization or a comparison group; after the group is given a pretest, the researcher introduces an intervention and then administers a posttest to examine changes between pretest and posttest scores

3. Use of pre-experimental designs is limiting because the researcher cannot determine cause-and-effect relationships and may be unable to rule out alternative explanations for the effect detected in the study

E. Nonexperimental designs

1. In a *nonexperimental design,* the researcher collects data without making changes or introducing an intervention

   a. It is an efficient and effective way of collecting a large amount of information about a problem in a realistic setting

   b. This type of design allows the researcher to investigate complex relationships among variables and to develop a foundation for future experimental studies

2. The researcher may use this type of design when the independent variable cannot be manipulated or should not be manipulated because of ethical considerations or when use of a true experimental or quasi-experimental design is impractical, undesirable, or inappropriate

3. Nonexperimental designs can be classified according to three types

   a. A *correlational design* is typically used to examine the relationship between two variables to see if, when one variable changes, the other variable also changes

   b. An *ex post facto design* is typically used to investigate the effect on the dependent variable after a change in the independent variable has occurred naturally; the researcher may use comparison groups in this type of design

   c. A *descriptive design* is typically used to observe, describe, or document aspects of a situation; this type of design does not concern the relationship between variables

4. Use of nonexperimental designs is limiting for two reasons

   a. The researcher cannot establish cause-and-effect relationships or determine why the variables respond as they do

   b. The researcher also may be unable to rule out alternative explanations for the effects detected in the study and may have difficulty interpreting the findings (see *Quantitative research designs,* pages 170 and 171)

CHECKLIST
Quantitative research designs

Use the following questions to critique the quantitative research design used in a study.

	Yes	No
General questions		
• Is the most appropriate design used for the research problem?	☐	☐
• Does the design flow from the purpose statement, literature review, theoretical framework, and hypothesis?	☐	☐
• Is the design realistic?	☐	☐
• Does the researcher use control methods to enhance internal and external validity?	☐	☐
• If a stronger design could have been used, does the researcher justify use of the weaker design?	☐	☐
• Are the major limitations of the selected design considered when interpreting the results?	☐	☐
True experimental design		
• Was a true experimental design used?	☐	☐
• Does the design address a cause-and-effect relationship?	☐	☐
• Is the researcher's use of manipulation, control, and randomization clear?	☐	☐
• Is the intervention described in detail?	☐	☐
• Are any alternative explanations for the results presented?	☐	☐
• Are the findings generalizable to the larger population?	☐	☐
Quasi-experimental and pre-experimental designs		
• Was a quasi-experimental or pre-experimental design used?	☐	☐
• Could the researcher have used a true experimental design instead?	☐	☐
• Were the most common threats to the internal and external validity of the study identified?	☐	☐
• Have all possible alternative explanations been satisfactorily discounted?	☐	☐
• Is the intervention described in detail?	☐	☐
Nonexperimental design		
• Was a nonexperimental design used?	☐	☐

Quantitative research designs (continued)

Nonexperimental design (continued)	Yes	No
• Is the design appropriate for the study?	☐	☐
• Does the researcher discuss the findings in a manner congruous with the design?	☐	☐
• Does the researcher attempt to infer cause-and-effect relationships?	☐	☐
• Does the researcher discuss threats to internal and external validity?	☐	☐
• Are alternative explanations addressed?	☐	☐

♦ III. Qualitative research designs

A. General information

  1. Qualitative research designs, relatively new to nursing research, provide insight, meaning, and understanding about a subject's experiences

  2. The researcher typically conducts a literature review after the data collection and analysis to avoid being influenced by preconceived expectations

  3. Intuition and empathy play key roles in qualitative research; the researcher typically becomes closely involved with the subjects in an attempt to understand their thoughts and ideas and must develop and cultivate intuitive and empathic feelings to prompt further dialogue

  4. Qualitative research designs have five primary purposes
     a. Describing phenomena
     b. Generating hypotheses
     c. Illustrating the meanings of relationships
     d. Understanding relationships
     e. Developing, refining, or expanding theory

  5. Concepts important to qualitative research designs include gestalt, bracketing, and intuiting
     a. *Gestalt* refers to the clustering of knowledge about a particular phenomenon into linked ideas to enhance meaning; qualitative research forms new gestalts to generate new theories
     b. *Bracketing* refers to the putting aside of what is known about a phenomenon to allow the researcher to observe it without preconceptions and to form new gestalts

      c. *Intuiting* refers to the process of examining the phenomenon being studied; this requires the researcher's concentration and complete absorption to focus on the area of interest

  6. Qualitative research designs can be classified into six major categories: phenomenologic, grounded theory, ethnographic, historical, philosophical inquiry, and critical social theory

B. Phenomenologic research design

  1. *Phenomenologic research* is based on the belief that no single reality exists and that individuals have separate and unique realities

  2. This design can enhance understanding through real-life experiences as described by participating subjects or informants; the researcher attempts to derive meaning by perceiving through the subject's reality

  3. The researcher identifies the phenomenon or experience to be explored and formulates one or more research questions; subjects are chosen based on their willingness to share personal experiences and feelings

  4. The researcher may use a combination of strategies to collect the data; data collection and analysis may occur simultaneously (see Chapters 21 and 22 for further details on data collection and analysis)

  5. Throughout the study, the researcher focuses on the actual experience, including which aspects of the experience the subjects perceive to be important and which changes or outcomes result from the experience

  6. Study findings may be described from the subjects' viewpoints

  7. Important considerations include maintaining a relaxed environment to elicit feelings about an experience and using bracketing and intuiting throughout the study

C. Grounded theory research design

  1. *Grounded theory research* is used to generate new theory from data collected without the aid of a pre-existing theory as a framework

  2. The researcher, who uses a combination of inductive and deductive reasoning, must remain open-minded about the findings

  3. This type of design is most useful in studying areas that have not been previously researched or in gaining a new viewpoint in known areas

  4. Intuiting plays an important role in grounded theory research

  5. Unlike the systematically arranged steps of other types of research, the steps in grounded theory research occur simultaneously; the researcher typically observes situations, collects data, organizes the data, and analyzes the data at the same time

  6. The researcher collects data through observations, interviews, or examination of pre-existing records and frequently relies on handwritten notes and tape recordings as a means of recording the data

7. The researcher attempts to collect data from as many diverse sources as possible to understand the situation fully; amassed data may be voluminous

8. The researcher analyzes the data using the constant comparative method (see chapter 22 for further information)

D. Ethnographic research design
1. *Ethnographic research* evolved from anthropology and involves the study of individuals or artifacts in a natural or real setting

2. Ethnographic research is primarily used to describe culture and is particularly helpful in the study of specific lifestyles or cultural phenomena from the subjects' viewpoints

3. The goal is to understand the insiders' (emic) view, which is compared and contrasted with the outsiders' (etic) view

4. In this type of research, the researcher becomes totally involved in the setting during data collection in an attempt to understand the daily life of the individual or group being studied but must maintain objectivity to avoid being assimilated into the culture or group

5. At the beginning of an ethnographic study, the researcher identifies the culture or group to be studied as well as significant variables within the culture or group, then conducts a literature review to learn as much as possible about what is already known about the culture or group

6. After gaining access to the culture or group, the researcher becomes immersed in the culture and tries to gain the confidence and support of individuals who are willing to explain cultural phenomena

7. Because extensive note taking is required during data collection, the researcher relies on intuition to determine which data to gather

8. The researcher typically uses direct observation to gather data; a description of the culture or group usually evolves from the data

9. The researcher develops theories to explain the relationships revealed by the data, which may lead to the formation of new hypotheses

E. Historical research design
1. *Historical research,* the careful examination and analysis of data from the past, is used to provide an understanding of the effect of the past on present and future events

2. This type of design is primarily based on the study of written materials; however, oral reports, photographs, films, and other artifacts also serve as sources of information

3. At the beginning of an historical study, the researcher formulates an idea, then clearly defines and narrows it to ensure that a search for related materials is realistic; afterward, the researcher develops general research questions to guide the study

4. After conducting a literature review, the researcher identifies and locates available sources, such as in private archives or libraries

5. After collecting the data, the researcher evaluates the information using external and internal criticism
   a. *External criticism* determines the data's genuineness and authenticity (validity)
   b. *Internal criticism* determines the data's truth and accuracy (reliability)
6. Collection of data may take months or years and may not have an obvious end
7. In analyzing the data, the researcher must clarify any conflicting evidence and decide which data to accept or reject as part of the findings
8. The written research report may be in the form of a biography or chronology, or it may focus on a particular issue

F. Philosophical inquiry research design
1. *Philosophical inquiry research* is conducted to debate issues or develop theories; analysis is used to examine the nature of values, ethics, and knowledge
2. The researcher uses inquiry and analysis to examine an issue from all perspectives
3. Philosophical questions guide the research, with data collection and analysis occurring simultaneously; answers generate additional questions that result in further analysis, creating a cyclical process
4. The researcher often discusses the analysis of questions and answers with colleagues
5. Reports focus on the conclusions of the analysis rather than on the methodology used
6. There are three types of philosophical inquiry
   a. Foundational inquiry examines the foundations of a science
   b. Philosophical analysis examines meanings
   c. Ethical analysis examines morality

G. Critical social theory research design
1. *Critical social theory research* is based on the belief that most societies function within patterns of domination and inhibit personal growth of individuals; certain societal facts are taken for granted and are not questioned or disputed
2. The researcher tries to understand how people develop symbolic meanings and tries to expose the constraints that impede free and equal participation in society
3. Using the structures of society, the researcher exposes issues of privilege, exploitation, and oppression to facilitate liberation and authenticity
4. Social structures of interest to nurses include images of women, health care delivery, families, and minorities
5. Feminist research uses critical social theory methods (see *Qualitative research designs*)

CHECKLIST
Qualitative research designs

Use the following questions to critique the qualitative research design used in a study.

	Yes	No
General questions		
• Does the research question seem to explore, describe, or expand knowledge about the phenomenon of interest?	☐	☐
• Is the most appropriate design used for the study?	☐	☐
• Has the research question been previously researched?	☐	☐
• Is the research question congruous with the philosophical basis of holism?	☐	☐
• Does evidence suggest that the researcher used bracketing and intuiting to form new gestalts about the phenomenon?	☐	☐
Phenomenologic research design		
• Does the study examine the phenomenon from the subject's or informant's perspective?	☐	☐
• Is the researcher an active participant in the subject's world?	☐	☐
• Has the researcher attempted to seek out individuals who are willing to share their feelings about the experience?	☐	☐
• Were the data collection methods appropriate?	☐	☐
• Did data collection and analysis occur simultaneously?	☐	☐
• Were the results described from the subject's or informant's viewpoint?	☐	☐
Grounded theory research design		
• Is the study phenomenon clearly identified?	☐	☐
• Has the phenomenon been previously researched?	☐	☐
• Is the researcher offering a fresh viewpoint on a familiar topic of interest?	☐	☐
• Does the researcher attempt to develop a theory about the phenomenon?	☐	☐
• Are data collection and recording methods appropriate for the situation?	☐	☐
• Does evidence suggest that the data were collected from as many sources as possible?	☐	☐
• Has the researcher collected, organized, and analyzed the data simultaneously?	☐	☐

(continued)

Qualitative research designs (continued)

	Yes	No
Ethnographic research design		
• Is the study conducted in a natural setting?	☐	☐
• Is the researcher totally involved in the setting during data collection?	☐	☐
• Does the researcher attempt to understand the subject's or informant's (emic) view and to describe the culture?	☐	☐
• Did the researcher become part of the culture?	☐	☐
• Did the researcher maintain objectivity?	☐	☐
• Did the researcher obtain the support and confidence of the subjects?	☐	☐
• Were data collection methods appropriate for the situation?	☐	☐
Historical research design		
• Does the study attempt to provide an understanding of how the past has influenced present or possible future events?	☐	☐
• Has the researcher clearly defined and narrowed the topic being studied?	☐	☐
• Were historical materials adequately analyzed and all possible sources of data explored?	☐	☐
• Has the researcher subjected the data to external and internal criticism?	☐	☐
• Did the researcher reconcile conflicting data and provide a valid rationale for drawing conclusions based on the study's findings?	☐	☐
Philosophical inquiry research design		
• Does the research debate an issue or examine the nature of values, ethics, or knowledge?	☐	☐
• Has the researcher analyzed the issue from all perspectives?	☐	☐
• Did the researcher use philosophical questions to guide the study?	☐	☐
• Did data collection and analysis occur simultaneously?	☐	☐
• Did the researcher focus on the conclusions of the analysis?	☐	☐
Critical social theory research design		
• Does the research explore a facet of society in which there are patterns of domination?	☐	☐

Qualitative research designs (continued)

Critical social theory research design *(continued)*	Yes	No
• Has the researcher exposed constraints that impede free and equal participation in society?	☐	☐
• Does the researcher seek to facilitate liberation and authenticity?	☐	☐

♦ IV. Other research designs

A. General information

    1. Other research designs may be used with quantitative or qualitative designs to provide the researcher with additional guidance

    2. Other commonly used research designs include cross-sectional, longitudinal, retrospective, prospective, survey, methodological, case study, secondary analysis, meta-analysis, and evaluation

B. Cross-sectional research designs

    1. A *cross-sectional research design* involves the simultaneous collection of data from different subjects at different stages of the same phenomenon to provide a total representation of the phenomenon

    2. This type of design is typically used in conjunction with a nonexperimental research design

    3. A cross-sectional design has three major advantages

        a. The design is practical and relatively manageable

        b. The researcher can use time efficiently and collect voluminous data economically

        c. Maturation is eliminated as a threat to internal validity

    4. A cross-sectional design also has three limitations

        a. The design structure may imply that differences between groups of subjects are attributable to time rather than generational variances

        b. Several alternative explanations may account for the observed differences

        c. The researcher cannot perform a detailed analysis of the interrelationships among the phenomena being studied

C. Longitudinal research designs

    1. A *longitudinal research design* involves the collection of data from the same subjects over time to provide information on changes or trends

    2. This type of design is typically used in conjunction with a nonexperimental research design

SEARCHING THE WEB
Qualitative research

A listing of qualitative research resources on the Internet can be found at
www.chass.ucr.edu/csbsr/qualitative.html.

3. Longitudinal designs can be classified into three types
   a. In a *panel study*, the researcher collects data from the same sample of subjects at two or more times
   b. In a *trend study*, the researcher collects data from different samples of subjects from the same population at two or more times
   c. In a *follow-up study*, the researcher collects data from the same sample of subjects, usually at a later time
4. A longitudinal design has four major advantages
   a. The design is useful in studying the interrelationships among variables over time
   b. The researcher can more accurately study changes that occur over time
   c. The timing of phenomena can be more easily determined
   d. The subjects can serve as their own controls
5. A longitudinal design also has three major limitations
   a. Loss of subjects (mortality) is a common threat to internal validity
   b. Data collection may be expensive and time-consuming
   c. Several alternative explanations may account for observed differences

D. Retrospective research designs
   1. A *retrospective research design* involves the collection of data about subjects' pasts (antecedent factors) to determine which factors, if any, precipitated or contributed to a current phenomenon
   2. This type of design, basically epidemiologic in nature, is typically used in conjunction with a nonexperimental (specifically, ex post facto) research design
   3. A retrospective design makes the researcher's work easier and more efficient in three areas
      a. The collection of voluminous data
      b. The exploration of complex relationships
      c. The generation of hypotheses that might provide a foundation for future experimental studies
   4. A retrospective design also has three major limitations
      a. The researcher cannot establish direct cause-and-effect relationships

b. Many alternative explanations for results cannot be ruled out

c. Findings may be difficult to interpret because the variables may be interrelated in complex ways

E. Prospective research designs

1. A *prospective research design* involves tracking subjects to observe for a phenomenon whose presumed cause has been identified

2. The purpose of a prospective design is to attempt to establish a stronger case for a cause-and-effect relationship

3. This type of design, basically epidemiologic in nature, may be used in conjunction with experimental, quasi-experimental, or nonexperimental research designs

4. A prospective design has three major advantages

   a. Questions involving the timing of events are easily resolved, because the independent variable can be manipulated to later observe for the dependent variable

   b. There is an increased likelihood that samples are representative of the population

   c. The researcher can impose controls that help rule out alternative explanations for the observed effects

5. A prospective design also has four major limitations

   a. The design typically is costly and time-consuming

   b. Loss of subjects is a threat to internal validity

   c. Alternative explanations for the observed results are possible if the research is quasi-experimental or nonexperimental

   d. A large sample of subjects is needed to conduct the study

F. Survey research designs

1. A *survey research design* involves data collection from a sample of subjects to examine the opinions, attitudes, behaviors, or characteristics of the population

2. A survey is similar to a *census* except that in a census, the researcher collects data from each member of the population

3. Data collection methods used in survey research include face-to-face interviews, telephone interviews, and written questionnaires

   a. *Face-to-face interviews* are the most effective means of conducting a survey because of the quality and amount of information obtained; however, they require much planning, interview training, and time

   b. *Telephone interviews* are typically an easy approach to collecting much information rapidly; however, subjects may be uncooperative and unresponsive

   c. *Questionnaires* are self-administered surveys that provide clear, simple, and unambiguous answers about subject characteristics; although economical and easily distributed through the mail, questionnaires may have a low return rate

4. A survey design has three major advantages
    a. The researcher can easily obtain voluminous data from many subjects
    b. The researcher can reach many populations and cover a wide range of topics
    c. The design's methodology can be easily stated so that the research is easier to evaluate and replicate
5. A survey design also has five major limitations
    a. Subjects may be reluctant to share certain information about themselves
    b. The information obtained tends to be superficial
    c. The researcher cannot draw cause-and-effect conclusions
    d. The survey may require much time and money
    e. Especially with questionnaires, a low response rate is possible

G. Methodological research designs
1. A *methodological research design* involves the development, testing, and evaluation of research instruments to develop reliable and valid research measures
2. This type of design, which is primarily concerned with the means by which researchers collect, organize, and analyze data, may be used with experimental, quasi-experimental, or nonexperimental designs
3. The researcher using a methodological design must be knowledgeable about PSYCHOMETRIC PROPERTIES
4. Methodological studies are particularly important in new fields, such as nursing research, that focus on complex, intangible phenomena
5. A methodological design has three major advantages
    a. The researcher can provide reliable and valid instruments greatly needed by other nursing researchers
    b. Newly discovered or invented instruments are immediately applicable
    c. The study can provide direction for other substantive research
6. A methodological design also has two major limitations
    a. Such studies are typically time-consuming and may become a researcher's lifework
    b. The new instrument may require many revisions with subsequent testing before it can be used by other researchers

H. Case study research designs
1. A *case study research design* involves the detailed investigation of an individual, group, or institution to understand which variables are important to the subject's history, development, or care
2. The researcher typically focuses on understanding why the subject thinks, behaves, or develops in a particular manner

3. A case study design has two major advantages
   a. The researcher may obtain detailed information about the subject, insight into complex relationships, and direction for future research
   b. The study can be conducted over time
4. A case study design also has three major limitations
   a. The researcher's familiarity with the subject makes objectivity difficult
   b. The results lack generalizability
   c. Cause-and-effect relationships cannot be determined

I. Secondary analysis research designs
   1. A *secondary analysis research design* involves further examination of previously collected data
   2. Variables not analyzed in an original research study are prime targets for a secondary analysis
   3. A secondary analysis design can be a powerful research tool if the researcher uses two or more sets of data with comparable variables
   4. A secondary analysis design has three major advantages
      a. The research can be efficiently and economically conducted
      b. The researcher can bypass the data collection phase
      c. Data are not wasted
   5. A secondary analysis design also has three major limitations
      a. The data may not contain all the information desired for analysis
      b. The researcher runs the risk of using inaccurate data
      c. Data relevant to the research topic may be difficult or impossible to find

J. Meta-analysis research designs
   1. A *meta-analysis research design* involves the merging of findings from several studies that have examined the same variables to integrate the findings and enhance their total contribution
   2. In a meta-analysis study, the researcher calculates a statistic (EFFECT SIZE) for the dependent variable of each study
   3. A meta-analysis design has three major advantages
      a. The researcher can integrate voluminous data objectively
      b. The researcher may discover new patterns and relationships that might otherwise have gone unnoticed
      c. Information obtained may be used in theory and future research development
   4. A meta-analysis design also has three major limitations
      a. Studies may be combined that conceptually do not belong together
      b. The results may be biased toward studies with only significant findings, because unpublished data probably will not be included

(Text continues on page 184.)

CHECKLIST
Miscellaneous research designs

Use the following questions to critique a miscellaneous research design in a study.

	Yes	No
Cross-sectional research design		
• Does the use of a cross-sectional approach seem appropriate?	☐	☐
• Were the data collected from all subjects at one time?	☐	☐
• Is a nonexperimental design used?	☐	☐
• Does the researcher identify alternative explanations for the results?	☐	☐
Longitudinal research design		
• Does the use of a longitudinal research design seem appropriate?	☐	☐
• Do the number of data collection points and the time intervals between data collections seem appropriate for the study?	☐	☐
• Was a panel, trend, or follow-up study used?	☐	☐
• Is a nonexperimental design used?	☐	☐
• Does the researcher identify alternative explanations for the results?	☐	☐
• Does the researcher address the problem of subject loss (mortality)?	☐	☐
Retrospective research design		
• Does the use of a retrospective research design seem appropriate?	☐	☐
• Has the researcher attempted to determine which past factors might have precipitated the present phenomenon?	☐	☐
• Does the study use a nonexperimental design?	☐	☐
• Does the researcher suggest hypotheses that could be tested in future research studies?	☐	☐
• Does the researcher identify alternative explanations for the results?	☐	☐
Prospective research design		
• Does a prospective research design seem appropriate for the study?	☐	☐
• Are selected subjects followed over time and observed for the occurrence of the phenomenon of interest?	☐	☐
• Does the researcher impose controls to rule out alternative explanations for the results obtained?	☐	☐

Miscellaneous research designs (continued)

	Yes	No
Prospective research design *(continued)*		
• Does the study use an experimental, a quasi-experimental, or a nonexperimental design?	☐	☐
Survey research design		
• Does the study lend itself to a survey?	☐	☐
• Was an appropriate data collection approach used?	☐	☐
• Was it the best one for the problem?	☐	☐
• Does the researcher clearly describe the contents of the survey and the methodology used?	☐	☐
• Does the researcher infer cause-and-effect relationships?	☐	☐
• Is the response rate specified?	☐	☐
• Does the researcher offer alternative explanations for the findings?	☐	☐
Methodological research design		
• Is the development of a reliable and valid instrument the focus?	☐	☐
• Does the study identify and define the concept to be measured?	☐	☐
• Are the results of reliability and validity tests reported?	☐	☐
Case study research design		
• Does the research involve a detailed investigation of an individual, a group, or an institution?	☐	☐
• Are the data collection methods clearly described and appropriate?	☐	☐
• Does the researcher overgeneralize the findings?	☐	☐
Secondary analysis research design		
• Does the researcher identify the source of data used for the secondary analysis?	☐	☐
• Is the purpose of the analysis specified?	☐	☐
• Does a secondary analysis seem appropriate for the study?	☐	☐
Meta-analysis research design		
• Does the researcher integrate findings from several research studies?	☐	☐
• Has the researcher attempted to obtain all research (published and unpublished) related to the variables of interest?	☐	☐

(continued)

Miscellaneous research designs (continued)

Meta-analysis research design *(continued)*	Yes	No
• Is the effect size for each study calculated?	☐	☐
• Does the researcher describe the study's limitations?	☐	☐
• Does the researcher overgeneralize the findings?	☐	☐
Evaluation research design		
• Does the research involve a detailed evaluation of a program?	☐	☐
• Is the evaluation clearly formative or summative?	☐	☐
• Does the research avoid bias in presenting the findings?	☐	☐
• Does the study use an experimental, a quasi-experimental, or a nonexperimental design?	☐	☐

    c. A research report may not contain sufficient information for the researcher to compute an effect size

K. Evaluation research designs
  1. An evaluation research design involves the collection of data to determine the effect of a program, policy, or intervention
  2. The type of evaluation may be formative or summative
    a. A formative or process evaluation is done to assess a program as it is being implemented
    b. A summative or outcome evaluation is done to assess the effect of a program after it is completed
  3. This type of design may be used in conjunction with experimental, quasi-experimental, or nonexperimental research designs
  4. An evaluation design has three major advantages
    a. The research can determine which method of care is best
    b. Studies can determine the cost-effectiveness of a program
    c. Data can validate that objectives have been met
  5. An evaluation design has two major limitations
    a. Objectivity may be difficult if the researcher was involved in program planning or implementation
    b. Findings may result in programs being eliminated (see *Miscellaneous Research Designs,* pages 182 to 184.)

Points to Remember

♦ The research design is the researcher's overall plan for obtaining answers to the research problem; choosing a research design is a major research decision.

♦ Qualitative research designs are based on holism, which focuses on the study of the total experience; quantitative research designs are based on reductionism, which focuses on the study of parts.

♦ Common threats to internal validity include history, maturation, testing, instrumentation, mortality, and selection bias.

♦ Common threats to external validity include adequacy of the population sample and environmental characteristics.

♦ True experimental research designs offer the greatest control over variables.

♦ Cross-sectional research designs collect data at one time; longitudinal research designs collect data several times.

♦ Retrospective research designs attempt to identify factors in a subject's past that might have precipitated a current phenomenon; prospective research follows a subject over time to observe for an effect whose presumed cause has been identified.

Study Questions

To evaluate your understanding of this chapter, answer the following questions in the space provided; compare your responses with the correct answers in appendix B, pages 237 to 244.

1. What is the difference between quantitative and qualitative research?

   _____

   _____

2. What are six threats to internal validity? _____

   _____

   _____

3. What are the characteristics of a true experimental design? _____

   _____

   _____

4. What are six major categories of a qualitative research design?

_____

_____

5. What is the difference between cross-sectional and longitudinal research designs?_____

_____

6. Which data collection methods are used in survey research designs?

_____

_____

7. Which research design involves the development, testing, and evaluation of research instruments? _____

_____

CRITICAL THINKING AND APPLICATION EXERCISES

1. Consider the research question, "What is it like to care for a spouse who has terminal cancer?" Which research design would be most appropriate?

2. Consider the research question, "Will postoperative patients who are transferred from the recovery room to the ICU for one day have fewer complications than patients who are transferred directly to the surgery floor?" Which research design would be most appropriate?

3. Read an experimental or quasi-experimental research article. Use the checklist on pages 170 and 171 to critique the research design.

4. Read a nonexperimental research article. Use the checklist on pages 170 and 171 to critique the research design.

5. Read a qualitative research article. Use the checklist on pages 175 to 177 to critique the research design.

20

Sampling Techniques

LEARNING OBJECTIVES

After studying this chapter, you should be able to:

♦ Define *population*.

♦ Identify the factors to consider when selecting a sample.

♦ Outline the steps used in selecting a sample.

♦ Discuss the four types of probability sampling techniques: simple random, stratified random, cluster, and systematic.

♦ Describe the four types of nonprobability sampling techniques: convenience, quota, purposive, and network.

♦ Compare and contrast probability and nonprobability sampling techniques.

♦ State the criteria for critiquing sampling techniques.

CHAPTER OVERVIEW

This chapter considers factors related to sampling techniques, defines sampling terms, and addresses sample size. It also lists the steps in selecting a sample, and describes types of probability and nonprobability samples. Pertinent questions to consider when critiquing sampling techniques are listed.

♦ I. Introduction

A. The following terms are commonly used in sampling

1. *Population*—entire group of ELEMENTS that meets a well-defined set of eligibility criteria; a population may consist of people, animals, objects, words, or events
2. *Eligibility criteria*—descriptors chosen by the researcher to define which elements should be included in or excluded from the population
3. *Sampling*—process of selecting a portion of the population to represent the entire population
4. *Sample*—subset of elements from the population
5. *Representative sample*—group of elements whose characteristics closely match those of the population
6. *Stratum*—mutually exclusive segment of the population (subpopulation) based on one or more characteristics, such as race or sex; strata are used to improve the representativeness of a sample
7. *Bias*—overrepresentation or underrepresentation of some segment or characteristic of a population in a research study; often happens with nonprobability samples
8. *Sampling frame*—list of all the elements in the population
9. *Sampling error*—difference between population values and sample values; the larger the sampling error, the less representative the sample is of the population

B. Sampling is used by researchers because it is an economical and efficient means of collecting data and because collecting data from the entire population usually is not necessary or feasible

C. The sampling technique, integral to the research, may affect the study's outcome
1. The criteria used to define the population affect the generalizability of the findings
2. The use of a sample that exhibits HOMOGENEITY with respect to key variables may result in bias, a potential threat to the study's external validity
3. The use of a sample that does not reflect the same variations as that of the population may lead to inconclusive findings

D. The researcher typically determines the sample size before collecting data

E. The researcher should consider several factors when selecting a sample: the type of sampling, the HETEROGENEITY of the variables being investigated, frequency of occurrence of the variable of interest, and the cost

F. Using the largest sample possible is usually best
1. Generally, the larger the sample, the more representative it will be
2. At least 10, but preferably 20 to 30, subjects should be selected for every variable or subset of data

CHECKLIST

Sampling techniques

Use the following questions to critique the sampling technique used in a study.

	Yes	No
• Is the population identified?	☐	☐
• Are the eligibility criteria specified?	☐	☐
• Are the sample selection techniques adequately described so that the sampling procedure can be replicated?	☐	☐
• Is a probability or nonprobability sampling technique used?	☐	☐
• Is the sample representative of the population?	☐	☐
• If any biases were introduced by the sampling technique, has the researcher identified them?	☐	☐
• Are the characteristics and size of the sample described?	☐	☐
• Is the sample size sufficient?	☐	☐
• Can the results be generalized to the population from which the sample was drawn?	☐	☐

   3. The researcher may be able to estimate the sample size needed using a statistical procedure known as POWER ANALYSIS
   4. Qualitative designs typically require much smaller samples than quantitative

G. Seven steps are involved in sampling
   1. Identifying and defining the population
   2. Delineating the accessible portion of the population
   3. Deciding how to choose the sample
   4. Determining the sample size, using power analysis if possible
   5. Obtaining permission from the human subjects committee or institutional review board to conduct the study
   6. Recruiting the subjects and obtaining informed consent
   7. Estimating the representativeness of the sample

H. The two basic sampling techniques used in nursing research are probability (RANDOM) sampling and nonprobability (nonrandom) sampling (see *Sampling techniques*)

♦ **II. Probability (random) sampling**

A. General information

1. Probability sampling involves the selection of elements from the population using random procedures in which each element of the population has an equal and independent chance of being chosen

2. Probability sampling is the only method of obtaining a representative sample, because the use of random techniques eliminates the possibility of researcher bias on a conscious and an unconscious level

3. When using probability sampling, the researcher can estimate the degree of sampling error

4. Probability sampling is important to the use of most statistical tests

5. Probability sampling, although preferred, has drawbacks

   a. It is expensive and inconvenient

   b. It may be impractical or unnecessary for certain studies

   c. The researcher has no guarantee that all randomly chosen subjects will participate in the study

6. Probability sampling can be further classified into four types: simple random, stratified random, cluster (multi-stage), and systematic

B. Simple random sampling

1. *Simple random sampling* allows the researcher to select elements randomly from a sampling frame

2. Typically, the researcher lists all of the elements of the population, numbers the elements consecutively, then uses a table of random numbers to draw the sample

3. Using this technique eliminates the possibility of researcher bias and guarantees that differences in sample characteristics are attributable to chance

4. Using this technique does not necessarily guarantee that the sample will be representative; however, the probability of choosing a non-representative sample decreases as the sample size increases

5. Researchers rarely use this technique because it is time-consuming and inefficient and because obtaining a complete list of every element in a population may be impossible

C. Stratified random sampling

1. *Stratified random sampling* involves the random selection of elements from two or more strata of the population to obtain a greater degree of representativeness

2. When using this technique, the researcher must divide the population into homogeneous strata, then randomly select the sample following the same steps used in simple random sampling (see above)

3. Using this technique guarantees the representation of different segments of the population and allows the researcher to oversample

from a small stratum to adjust for its underrepresentation in the population

4. Using stratified random sampling may be time-consuming, and the researcher may have difficulty establishing a stratified sampling frame that includes all the necessary elements

D. Cluster (multi-stage) sampling

1. *Cluster sampling* involves the random sampling of elements from large groups (CLUSTERS) to successively smaller groups to narrow the sample to the smallest grouping possible

2. Typically, the researcher proceeds from the largest cluster (such as U.S. states) to progressively smaller clusters (such as counties, voting districts, and households) to arrive at the smallest element possible (such as male heads of households)

3. Cluster sampling is more economical and practical than simple or stratified random techniques, but it typically results in more sampling errors

E. Systematic sampling

1. *Systematic sampling* involves the random selection of subjects from the population based on a fixed SAMPLING INTERVAL (such as every 10th person in the sampling frame)

2. Most researchers prefer systematic sampling instead of simple random sampling because they can obtain the same results more efficiently and conveniently

3. Use of this technique may result in problems or questionable findings if the sampling frame is arranged so that a particular characteristic coincides with the sampling interval (for example, if every 10th person listed in the sampling frame is male)

♦ III. Nonprobability (nonrandom) sampling

A. General information

1. Nonprobability sampling involves the selection of elements from a population using nonrandom procedures

2. Nonprobability sampling techniques are typically less rigorous and less representative than probability sampling techniques

3. Most research samples are based on nonprobability sampling because these techniques are feasible, practical, and relatively inexpensive

4. The major disadvantage to using nonprobability sampling is the researcher's limited ability to generalize from the findings

5. Nonprobability sampling can be further classified into four types: convenience, quota, purposive (judgmental), and network (snowball)

SEARCHING THE WEB
Sampling in research

An eight-page tutorial on sampling in research can be found on the Internet at http://trochim.human.cornell.edu/tutorial/mugo/tutorial.htm.

B. Convenience (accidental) sampling
1. *Convenience sampling* involves the nonrandom selection of subjects based on their availability or convenient accessibility
2. Although easy to obtain, they are considered the weakest type of samples
3. Use of this technique may result in questionable findings, because the most available subjects may not be typical of the population in terms of the variables of interest
4. With convenience sampling, the risk of researcher bias is great and external validity is compromised

C. Quota sampling
1. *Quota sampling* involves the nonrandom selection of elements based on the identification of specific characteristics to increase the sample's representativeness
2. Similar to stratified random sampling, quota sampling is based on the identification of certain strata within the population and the proportional representation of each of those strata in the sample
3. Quota sampling helps to address the overrepresentation and underrepresentation of certain elements in the population
4. This technique contains an unknown degree of bias that affects external validity

D. Purposive (judgmental) sampling
1. *Purposive sampling* involves the nonrandom selection of elements based on the researcher's judgment and knowledge about the population
2. Purposive sampling is useful when a group of subjects is needed to participate in a pretest of newly developed instruments or when a group of experts is desirable to validate research information; it is frequently used with qualitative research designs
3. With purposive sampling, the risk of conscious and unconscious bias is great and the researcher's ability to generalize from the findings is limited

E. Network (snowball) sampling
1. Network sampling involves the nonrandom selection of elements based on social networks

2. When the researcher has found one subject who meets the criteria, that person is asked to help recruit or locate other subjects
3. This technique is used to obtain subjects difficult to locate, such as alcoholics, drug abusers, and criminals
4. With network sampling, the risk of bias is great because the subjects know each other

POINTS TO REMEMBER

♦ A population is the entire group of elements that meets the eligibility criteria; a sample is the subset of elements from the population being studied.

♦ Generally, the larger the sample, the more representative it will be of the population.

♦ A power analysis is typically the most accurate way to determine sample size.

♦ Simple random, stratified random, cluster, and systematic sampling are types of probability sampling techniques.

♦ Convenience, quota, purposive, and network sampling are types of non-probability sampling techniques.

♦ Nonprobability sampling techniques typically are more feasible, practical, and economical than probability sampling techniques but result in less representative samples.

STUDY QUESTIONS

To evaluate your understanding of this chapter, answer the following questions in the space provided; compare your responses with the correct answers in appendix B, pages 237 to 244.

1. What is a population? _____

_____

_____

2. What is the difference between probability and nonprobability sampling techniques? _____

_____

_____

3. What are four types of probability sampling? _____

_____

_____

4. What are four types of nonprobability sampling? _____

_____

_____

CRITICAL THINKING AND APPLICATION EXERCISES

1. Create a sampling frame consisting of 10 men and 10 women and their ages. Calculate the average age for this population of 20 people. Randomly draw samples of 2, 4, 6, 8, and 10 subjects. Compare the gender and average age of each sample to the population data. Consider how representativeness increases as the sample becomes larger.

2. Create a sampling frame consisting of 10 men and 10 women whose ages are between 30 and 40. Calculate the average age for this population of 20 people. Randomly draw samples of 2, 4, 6, 8, and 10 subjects. Compare the gender and average age of each sample to the population data. How did homogeneity affect representativeness of the sample?

3. A researcher is planning to study college students' attitudes about writing research reports and decides to approach students entering the university library and ask them to participate in the study. What type of sampling is being used? What better way could be used to obtain a sample?

4. Read a quantitative research article. Use the checklist on page 189 to critique the sampling technique.

5. Read a qualitative research article. Use the checklist on page 189 to critique the sampling technique.

Data Collection Methods and Measurement Techniques

CHAPTER OVERVIEW

This chapter outlines various data collection methods and measurement techniques. It discusses instrument reliability and validity as well as methods for determining reliability and validity, and it reviews nominal, ordinal, interval, and

195

ratio levels of measurement. Also discussed are questionnaires and interviews, scales, observation, and physiologic measures. Pertinent questions to consider when critiquing data collection methods and measurement techniques are listed.

♦ I. Introduction

A. *Data collection* is the process by which the researcher acquires subjects and collects the information needed to answer the research problem

B. Data collection allows the researcher to measure the variables in the study

C. Before collecting the data, the researcher must make a number of decisions
1. Which data to collect
2. How to collect the data
3. Who will collect the data
4. Where to collect the data
5. When to collect the data

D. The researcher may use various data collection methods to gather information, such as questionnaires, interviews, scales, observation, or physiologic measures (see *Data collection methods and measurement techniques*)

E. The researcher should base the selection of a data collection method on three concerns
1. The identified hypothesis or research question
2. The research design
3. The amount of information already known about the variables

F. The device used to collect the data is referred to as an *instrument* or a *tool*
1. Instruments facilitate variable observation and measurement
2. The researcher may rely on an existing instrument or may develop a new one to fit the study's needs
   a. Instrument development requires a high degree of research expertise, because the instrument must be reliable and valid
      (1) *Reliability* refers to the degree of consistency and accuracy with which an instrument measures a variable
      (2) *Validity* refers to the extent to which an instrument measures what it is designed to measure
      (3) An unreliable instrument cannot be valid, but a reliable instrument can be invalid
   b. An instrument is considered highly reliable if it demonstrates little variation with repeated measurements and has a high *true score* (little measurement error)
      (1) An instrument's reliability can be further defined according to its stability, internal consistency, and equivalence

CHECKLIST

Data collection methods and measurement techniques

Use the following questions to critique the data collection method used in a study.

	Yes	No
General questions		
• Is the data collection method clearly described?	☐	☐
• Is the appropriate method used for the research design and the population?	☐	☐
• Is the same data collection method used for all subjects?	☐	☐
• Does the researcher discuss the reliability and validity of the method used?	☐	☐
Questionnaires and interviews		
• Is the degree of structure consistent with the research question?	☐	☐
• Did the researcher use the appropriate method (questionnaire vs. interview) for the research design?	☐	☐
• Is the questionnaire or interview schedule sufficiently described to determine whether it covers the variable of interest?	☐	☐
• Did sufficient numbers of subjects respond?	☐	☐
• If an interview was used, were the interviewers trained?	☐	☐
Scales		
• Does the scale adequately cover the variables?	☐	☐
• Did the researcher use the most appropriate scale for collecting the data?	☐	☐
• If the researcher used a new scale, was it adequately pretested and refined?	☐	☐
• Does the researcher address the possibility of response-set biases?	☐	☐
Observation		
• Is the degree of structure imposed by the researcher consistent with the research question?	☐	☐
• Were the observers required to make any judgments about what they observed?	☐	☐
• Was an appropriate category system, checklist, or rating scale used?	☐	☐

(continued)

Data collection methods and measurement techniques (continued)

Observation *(continued)*	Yes	No
• Did the observer's presence affect the subjects' behavior?	☐	☐
• If time sampling or event sampling was used, did the sampling plan yield relevant behaviors?	☐	☐
Physiologic measures		
• Was the proper instrument used to obtain the measurements?	☐	☐
• If an invasive procedure was used, could a noninvasive procedure have yielded similar information?	☐	☐
• Did the instrument appear to have any effect on the variable being measured?	☐	☐
• Was the instrument reliable and valid for the variable of interest?	☐	☐

    (a) *Stability* refers to the extent to which the same results are obtained with repeated use of an instrument; stability is usually assessed by test-retest, which should be 0.70 or above

    (b) *Internal consistency* refers to the extent to which all parts of an instrument measure the same variable; internal consistency is usually assessed by Cronbach's alpha, which should be 0.70 or above

    (c) *Equivalence* refers to the extent to which different observers or different forms of an instrument yield the same results; equivalence is usually assessed by interrater reliability, which should be 0.80 or above

  (2) An instrument's validity can be further classified as content, concurrent, predictive, or construct

    (a) *Content validity* refers to the extent to which an instrument measures the variable's expected content; the researcher typically verifies content validity by conducting a literature review to determine which content should be covered and by asking experts to evaluate the instrument's representativeness of the content

    (b) *Concurrent validity* refers to the extent to which an instrument can accurately identify subjects who differ with respect to a given characteristic; the researcher typically validates concurrent validity by using the instrument in conjunction with a second instrument already known to be valid

SEARCHING THE WEB
Reliability versus validity

A five-page tutorial on the differences between reliability and validity can be found at http://trochim.human.cornell.edu/tutorial/colosi/colosi2.htm.

     (c) *Predictive validity* refers to the extent to which an instrument can accurately forecast characteristics; the researcher typically validates predictive validity by using the instrument, then comparing the results with some future outcome

     (d) *Construct validity* refers to the extent to which an individual actually possesses the characteristic being measured by the instrument; the researcher typically validates construct validity by using the KNOWN-GROUPS TECHNIQUE, hypothesis testing, convergent and divergent approaches, or factor analysis

♦ II. Measurement techniques

A. General information

  1. *Measurement,* integral to quantitative research, is the process by which the researcher assigns specific numbers to the collected data

  2. The researcher measures each variable of the collected data according to its magnitude or quantity

  3. Measurements are made based on two assumptions

    a. Everything exists in some amount, which can be measured

    b. Attributes of an object vary, and the variability can be expressed as a number that indicates how much of the attribute is present

  4. The researcher may use one of four levels of measurement (nominal, ordinal, interval, or ratio) when collecting data

  5. The researcher should always aim for the highest level of measurement possible; generally, the higher the level, the more information is available for analysis

    a. Data measured at one level may be downgraded to a lower level, but never advanced to a higher level

    b. The level of measurement affects the types of statistical analyses that can be performed on the collected data

B. Nominal level

  1. With the *nominal level* (the lowest level), the researcher assigns numbers to categorize specific characteristics of a variable (for example, in relation to marital status, 0 might represent single and 1, married)

2. The numbers do not have quantitative meaning and cannot be manipulated mathematically

3. The amount in each category can be counted and occurrence can be determined

4. Examples of nominal-level variables are gender, marital status, health status, and nursing specialty

C. Ordinal level

1. With the *ordinal level* (the second lowest level), the researcher assigns numbers to categories and sorts variables based on their relative rank

2. The intervals between the categories are not considered equal

3. The numbers have some quantitative meaning and can be manipulated mathematically but only to a limited degree

4. Examples of ordinal-level variables are ranking of height (tallest to shortest) and pain intensity (mild, moderate, or severe)

D. Interval level

1. With the *interval level* (the second highest level), the researcher assigns numbers to categories and ranks the variables according to equally spaced intervals

2. Interval-level measures do not have an ABSOLUTE ZERO POINT

3. The possibility of mathematical manipulations is greatly increased; addition and subtraction can be meaningfully calculated

4. Examples of interval-level variables are Fahrenheit and centigrade temperatures (see *Intervals versus ordinal levels*)

E. Ratio level

1. With the *ratio level* (the highest level), the researcher not only assigns numbers to categories and ranks the variables according to equally spaced intervals as in interval-level measurement, but also designates an absolute, meaningful zero

2. All mathematical manipulations, such as addition, subtraction, multiplication, and division, can be calculated

3. Examples of ratio-level variables are height, weight, time, and length

F. Measurement error

1. All measurements used in data collection are fallible; all results have some degree of error

2. All measured results contain a true score and an error component
   a. The *true score* is the value that would be obtained if the measurement instrument were perfect
   b. The *error component* is the difference between the true score and the measured score

3. Measurement error is the result of extraneous factors that distort the measured score

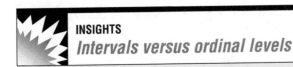

INSIGHTS
Intervals versus ordinal levels

Within nursing, controversy exists about the level of measurement assigned to scores from attitude scales and personality tests. Some researchers regard these measures as interval levels; others consider them to be ordinal. Because interval level data allow greater statistical analysis, many argue for the higher classification.

♦ III. Questionnaires and interviews

A. General information

1. Questionnaires and interviews are the most commonly used data collection methods in nursing research
2. Questions may be either closed-ended or open-ended
   a. CLOSED-ENDED QUESTIONS allow the subjects to choose appropriate answers from a predetermined list of responses; such questions facilitate analysis and ensure comparability of responses; although they are easy to administer, they are difficult to construct
   b. OPEN-ENDED QUESTIONS allow the subjects to respond in their own words; although they typically provide detailed information, they are time-consuming and sometimes difficult to analyze

B. Types of questionnaires and interviews

1. The questionnaire or interview schedule may be highly structured, totally unstructured, or semistructured
2. A *highly structured* questionnaire or interview schedule contains only predetermined questions and response options; subjects are asked to respond to the same questions in the same order, using the same set of response options
3. In a *totally unstructured* questionnaire or interview schedule, the researcher collects data with no preconceived plan of content or order of information to obtain; subjects are simply encouraged to relate their experiences; unstructured interviews are often used in qualitative research
4. *Semistructured* questionnaires and interview schedules contain some open-ended questions and some closed-ended questions, and a specific format for obtaining the information is followed

C. Advantages of questionnaires and interviews

1. Questionnaires are relatively efficient data collection methods in terms of money, time, and ease of administration
2. Questionnaires offer the possibility of subjects' anonymity

3. Interviews are associated with a high response rate and can be used with most subjects
4. Interviews allow the researcher to observe the subjects while they respond to questions, which may lead to more information

D. Disadvantages of questionnaires and interviews
1. Questionnaires may have a low response rate because the subjects can disregard or ignore the questionnaire
2. Questionnaires require subjects' ability to read, write, and comprehend questions to avoid misinterpretation
3. Interviews require considerable time and money and cannot offer subjects anonymity
4. Interviews introduce the possibility of bias because of interviewer-subject interaction
5. The reliability and validity of questionnaires and interviews depend on subjects' honest responses

♦ IV. Scales

A. General information
1. A scale is a commonly used data collection method in which the researcher asks subjects to rank variables on a continuum; it allows the researcher to distinguish quantitatively among subjects who differ with respect to the variables of interest
2. Researchers typically use scales to measure psychosocial variables, such as self-concept, personality traits, and attitudes

B. Types of scales
1. *Rating scales* require subjects to rate or rank a phenomenon at some point along a continuum that has been assigned a numerical value (for example, subjects might be asked to rate an object on a scale of 1 to 10, with 10 being the highest score)
2. *Likert scales,* the most commonly used scales in nursing research, are designed to elicit opinions or attitudes; subjects are asked to indicate how strongly they agree or disagree with a series of statements based on a 4- to 7-point scale
3. The *semantic differential scale* is used to measure attitudes or beliefs
   a. It consists of two opposite adjectives (such as "important" and "unimportant," or "weak" and "strong"), with a 7-point scale between them
   b. Subjects are asked to indicate the one point on the scale that describes their view of a variable of interest
4. *Guttman scales* consist of a group of four or five statements with which the subject is asked to agree or disagree; the statements relate to only one variable and are arranged in a hierarchy, so that the subject who agrees with the strongest statement of the group will probably agree with all of the other statements on the scale

2. All quantitative data analyses begin with descriptive statistics
   a. The extent to which the researcher relies on descriptive statistics depends on the type of research design
   b. For example, in exploratory or descriptive research designs, descriptive statistics are typically the only statistics used for data analysis; in other research designs, descriptive statistics are typically used to summarize the sample characteristics
3. Descriptive statistics can be classified into four categories: frequency distributions, measures of central tendency, measures of variability, and bivariate descriptive statistics
   a. *Frequency distribution* is the arrangement of all numerical values assigned to variables, from the lowest to the highest, along with a listing of the number of times each value was obtained; this arrangement is a useful way of organizing and summarizing data and can be used for analysis
      (1) Frequency distributions can be ungrouped (each value is listed separately) or grouped (values are organized according to ranges or intervals)
      (2) Frequency distributions may be displayed in table or graph form (see *Frequency distributions: Tables and graphs*, page 210)
      (3) When represented in graph form, frequency distributions are typically described in terms of their curved shape
         (a) They may be symmetrical (consisting of identical halves) or asymmetrical (containing off-center peaks and unequal sides or tails; asymmetrical curves, also known as skewed curves, can be positively or negatively skewed, depending on the direction in which the tail is pointing)
         (b) They may be unimodal (containing only one peak) or multimodal (containing two or more peaks)
         (c) A normal distribution curve (depicted by a bell-shaped curve that is symmetrical, unimodal, and not too peaked) represents the normal variations of a variable within a given population (50% of the values lie on the right half of the curve and 50% lie on the left half)
   b. *Measures of central tendency* are statistics that summarize the data into one representative value; they include the mode, the median, and the mean
      (1) The *mode* is the score or category that has the highest frequency or that occurs most often on a frequency distribution; it is typically used with nominal-level measures; the mode for the frequency distribution on page 210 is 24
      (2) The *median* is the number that lies midpoint in a distribution and divides the scores in half; because of its insensitivity to extreme values, the median is commonly the preferred

Frequency distributions: Tables and graphs

A frequency distribution—a systematic arrangement of numerical values, from the lowest to the highest, coupled with a tally of the number of times each value was obtained—may be illustrated in the form of a table or graph. Below are examples of various frequency distributions representing the raw test scores of a group of 50 students whose scores ranged from 20 to 30.

FREQUENCY TABLE

Raw scores	Tallies	Frequency	Percentage (%)
20	‖ ‖	4	8.0
21	‖	3	6.0
22	‖ ‖	4	8.0
23	‖ ‖	5	10.0
24	‖ ‖ ‖ ‖	9	18.0
25	‖ ‖ ‖	7	14.0
26	‖ ‖ ‖	6	12.0
27	‖ ‖	4	8.0
28	‖	3	6.0
29	‖	3	6.0
30	‖	2	4.0

HISTOGRAM

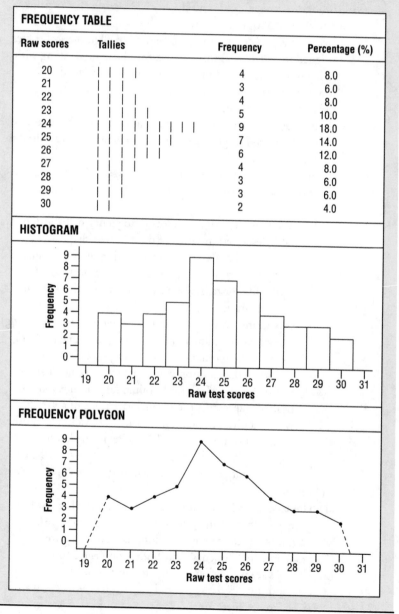

FREQUENCY POLYGON

measure of central tendency when the distribution is skewed; the median for the frequency distribution on page 210 is 24.5

(3) The *mean* is the arithmetic average of a distribution that can be used with only interval or ratio data; the mean, which is commonly symbolized as X or M, is the most commonly used measure of central tendency and the least likely to fluctuate widely from one sample to another sample drawn from the same population; the mean for the frequency distribution on page 210 is 24.64

c. *Measures of variability* are statistics that concern the degree to which the scores in a distribution are different from or similar to each other; the two most commonly used are the range and the standard deviation

(1) The *range* is the distance between the highest score and the lowest score in a distribution; the range for the frequency distribution on page 210 is 10

(2) The *standard deviation* is the most commonly used measure of variability; it indicates the average to which scores deviate from the mean; the standard deviation, commonly symbolized as *SD*, is an indication of the degree of error involved when the mean is used to describe a distribution; the standard deviation for the frequency distribution on page 210 is 2.686

(3) A normal distribution contains approximately three standard deviations above and below the mean; about 68% of all scores fall within one standard deviation of the mean, about 95% fall within two standard deviations of the mean, and about 99% fall within three standard deviations of the mean

d. *Bivariate (two-variable) descriptive statistics* are those derived from the simultaneous analysis of two variables to examine the relationships between the variables; the two most commonly used in quantitative analysis are contingency tables and correlation

(1) A *contingency table* allows the visual comparison of two or more categories of nominal- or ordinal-level data; typically, the data are in the form of numbers or percentages that appear within individual table cells

(2) *Correlation,* which may be descriptive or inferential, involves the use of a correlation coefficient (ranging from +1.00 to −1.00) to describe the relationship between two variables

(a) A correlation coefficient of 0 indicates that no relationship exists between the two variables

(b) A correlation coefficient between 0 and +1.00 indicates a positive relationship (as one variable increases, the other variable also increases)

(c) A correlation coefficient between 0 and −1.00 indicates a negative or inverse relationship (as one variable increases, the other variable decreases)

(d) The higher the absolute value of the coefficient, the stronger the relationship (for example, −0.75 indicates a stronger relationship than +0.25)

(e) The *product moment correlation coefficient,* known as the PEARSON *r*, is the most commonly used correlation procedure involving interval- or ratio-level data

C. Inferential statistics

1. *Inferential statistics* are numerical values used to draw conclusions about a population based on the characteristics of a population sample

2. Inferential statistics are based on the laws of probability

3. The underlying assumption is that only chance is responsible for variation among samples of the same population

4. Inferential statistics provide objective criteria for deciding whether a hypothesis should be accepted as true or rejected as false and for deciding which outcomes probably resulted from chance

5. An important factor in determining the degree to which chance affects the findings is the level of significance the researcher assigns to the findings

   a. The *level of significance* is a numerical value selected by the researcher before data collection to indicate the probability of erroneous findings being accepted as true; this value typically is selected as 0.01 or 0.05

   b. A 0.05 level of significance indicates that of 100 samples, the researcher would expect 5 samples to yield erroneous findings and 95 samples to yield accurate findings; a 0.01 level of significance indicates that of 100 samples, the researcher would expect 1 sample to yield erroneous findings and 99 samples to yield accurate findings

6. Because statistical inference is based on data from a sample rather than the entire population, there are two possible error types: type I error and type II error

   a. Type I error occurs when a true null hypothesis is rejected as false

   b. Type II error occurs when a false null hypothesis is accepted as true

7. Inferential statistical tests can be classified according to two types: parametric and nonparametric; parametric tests are more powerful and flexible than nonparametric tests and are preferred by most researchers

   a. *Parametric* tests focus on population parameters, require measurements on an interval or ratio level, and assume that the variables are normally distributed in the population

CHECKLIST
Quantitative data analysis

Use the following questions to critique the quantitative data analysis used in a study.

	Yes	No
• Does the research question or hypothesis lend itself to quantitative analysis?	☐	☐
• Was the level of measurement appropriate for the data collection tool?	☐	☐
• Were the statistical tests appropriate for the level of measurement?	☐	☐
• Have all frequencies, measures of central tendency, and measures of variability been reported?	☐	☐
• Was a statistical test performed for each research question or hypothesis?	☐	☐
• Did the researcher select an appropriate level of significance?	☐	☐
• If a parametric test was used, were the data measured on an interval or a ratio level? Were the variables normally distributed throughout the population?	☐	☐
• If a nonparametric test was used, could the researcher have used a more powerful parametric test?	☐	☐
• Did the researcher present a sufficient amount of information about the analyzed data and results to support the hypothesis or research question?	☐	☐
• Did the researcher use frequency distribution tables or graphs to summarize large amounts of data? Are they clearly labeled and consistent with the text?	☐	☐

  b. *Nonparametric* tests are not based on population parameters, use nominal- or ordinal-level data, and assume nothing about the distribution of the variables in the population

8. The most commonly used inferential statistical tests include the *t*-test, analysis of variance, chi-square analysis, Mann-Whitney *U*, Kruskal-Wallis, Wilcoxon signed-rank, correlation coefficient, simple linear regression, multiple regression, canonical correlation, analysis of covariance, multivariate analysis of variance, discriminant analysis, and path analysis (see *Quantitative data analysis*)

SEARCHING THE WEB
Information on inferential statistics

A learning package on inferential statistics can be found on the World Wide Web at www.cvgs.k12.va.us/DIGSTATS/inferent/lmain.htm. The menu takes you to activities related to *t*-test, ANOVA, correlation, regression, and two-way ANOVA (Factorial).

◆ III. Qualitative data analysis

  A. General information

    1. Qualitative data analysis relies on intuition and analytical reasoning to guide the organization, reduction, and clustering of data

    2. The researcher typically uses three strategies to analyze the data

      a. *Reduction* is the minute examination of voluminous narrative data that allows the researcher to deduce inherent meanings

      b. *Data display* is the organization of data using tables, graphs, and matrices

      c. *Conclusion drawing and verification* is the process whereby the researcher attaches meaning to the findings

    3. Many researchers use computers to help with data analysis

    4. Examples of computer programs available for analysis of qualitative data include Ethnograph, QUALPRO, Text Analysis Package, and HyperQual

    5. Qualitative data analysis is particularly challenging for three reasons

      a. The researcher has no systematic rules to guide the analysis and interpretation of data

      b. The researcher must devote much time and work to reading, organizing, and analyzing the data

      c. The findings cannot be briefly summarized (in fact, many analyses are published as books rather than as research articles)

    6. The researcher must develop an effective record-keeping and data retrieval system, either manually or on computer, in which all data are labeled, indexed, sorted, and filed

    7. The scientific rigor of qualitative analysis is judged by four criteria: credibility, auditability, fittingness, and confirmability

      a. Credibility is the truth of the findings as judged by informants and professionals

      b. Auditability is the adequacy of the information leading to the interpretation of the findings

      c. Fittingness is the inclusion of detail so that others can evaluate importance for practice

       d. Confirmability is implementation of standards that reflect credibility, auditability, and fittingness

    8. The researcher may use one of four methods to conduct qualitative data analysis: the constant comparative method, content analysis, analytical induction, or hermeneutical analysis

B. Constant comparative method

    1. The *constant comparative method* is a means of analyzing data collected through grounded theory in which the researcher collects and analyzes data simultaneously without the use of a pre-existing theory as an organizing framework

    2. In this type of analysis, which typically requires considerable time and the ability to think conceptually, the researcher attempts to discover patterns or social behaviors to form the basis of a relevant and useful theory that has the potential for generalizability

    3. To conduct a constant comparative analysis, the researcher first formulates a research question, then uses theoretical sampling to obtain data from various subjects and situations

    4. After obtaining the data, the researcher takes the following steps

       a. Establishes categories or codes based on the similarity or dissimilarity of the content

       b. Compares each incident with the category to determine if each incident fits

       c. Examines categories for uniformities and differences

       d. Reviews the literature to discover how the current research fits with existing research

       e. Discovers the overriding conceptual scheme that accounts for most of the relationships or patterns observed

       f. Sorts the data into a coherent whole that integrates all of the main ideas into a scheme

       g. Writes a report

C. Content analysis

    1. *Content analysis* involves the systematic and objective quantification of data to analyze the content of individual words, phrases, sentences, or themes

    2. Used with either oral or written data, content analysis is especially useful in historical research because of the efficient manner in which materials are used (see *Content analysis,* page 216)

    3. The researcher strives to maintain objectivity by having two people analyze the same data

    4. To conduct a content analysis, the researcher takes the following steps

       a. Identifies and selects the variables or concepts to be recorded and the unit of analysis (the word, phrase, sentence, or theme) to be used

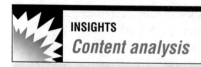

INSIGHTS
Content analysis

Because content analysis may involve counting coded information in the process of analyzing the data, some researchers do not consider it a qualitative technique. However, content analysis is used to examine the frequency, order, or intensity of words or phrases that are considered the focus of qualitative analysis.

    b. Formulates a coding and category system for classifying the units of analysis

    c. Develops definitions and illustrations to guide the coding of data into categories

    d. Analyzes the data by examining the coded information

    e. Draws conclusions

    f. Issues a report of the findings

D. Analytical induction

    1. *Analytical induction* involves searching for concepts and propositions in data that are applicable to all cases of the topic of interest or question being studied

    2. The researcher must carefully consider all aspects of the data, analyze each case separately, and compare each case to the others

    3. To conduct analytical induction, the researcher takes the following steps

        a. Defines the phenomenon to be analyzed

        b. Reviews the data

        c. Formulates a hypothetical explanation of the phenomenon

        d. Examines each case to see if the hypothesis applies

        e. Searches for negative cases (situations for which the hypothesis does not apply)

        f. Reformulates the hypothesis, as necessary

        g. Continues examining cases and reformulating the hypothesis until a universal pattern of relationships is identified and supported by the data

E. Hermeneutical analysis

    1. *Hermeneutical analysis,* sometimes called phenomenological-interpretive analysis, is a holistic approach to analysis that involves the examination and interpretation of field notes or interviews to understand the meanings and practices of people functioning as whole beings in specific situations

    2. Hermeneutical analysis is based on three assumptions

CHECKLIST
Qualitative data analysis

Use the following questions to critique the qualitative data analysis used in a study.

	Yes	No
• Was qualitative analysis appropriate for the research question and design?	☐	☐
• If any of the qualitative data were converted to quantitative data, was the level of quantification appropriate?	☐	☐
• Were the sources of data (such as observations or interviews) sufficient to yield a broad range of material for analysis?	☐	☐
• Did the researcher provide excerpts from the narrative material to demonstrate and substantiate the themes identified in the data?	☐	☐
• Did the researcher search for negative cases?	☐	☐
• Is the researcher's attempt to be objective evident?	☐	☐
• Is there evidence of credibility, auditability, fittingness, and confirmability?	☐	☐

      a. Language is used by individuals to communicate their ideas about reality

      b. The researcher's task is to uncover and understand the meanings embedded in communication

      c. The researcher must study experiences of daily life

3. The researcher typically analyzes the data to identify which aspects of specific behaviors or situations are important to the subject and the specific meanings the subject attaches to them

4. The researcher may use one of three approaches to conducting hermeneutical analysis

      a. *Thematic analysis* involves reading each interview to identify common themes

      b. *Analysis of exemplars* involves examining events taken from interviews to generate descriptions of situations and behaviors

      c. *Identification of a* PARADIGM CASE involves examining all cases to find similarities between the paradigm and the other cases (see *Qualitative data analysis*)

POINTS TO REMEMBER

♦ The purpose of data analysis is to impose order on a large amount of information so that conclusions can be made and communicated.

♦ Computers can be widely used in data analysis and have almost eliminated the need for manual statistical computations.

♦ Descriptive statistics include frequency distributions, measures of central tendency, measures of variability, and bivariate statistics.

♦ Commonly used inferential statistical tests include the *t*-test, analysis of variance, chi-square, Mann-Whitney *U*, Kruskal-Wallis, Wilcoxon signed-rank, correlation coefficient, simple linear regression, multiple regression, canonical correlation, analysis of covariance, multivariate analysis of variance, discriminant analysis, and path analysis.

♦ Qualitative data may be analyzed using the constant comparative method, content analysis, analytical induction, or hermeneutical analysis.

STUDY QUESTIONS

To evaluate your understanding of this chapter, answer the following questions in the space provided; compare your responses with the correct answers in appendix B, pages 237 to 244.

1. What is the purpose of data analysis? _____

_____

_____

2. Which type of data analysis uses numbers and statistical computations?

_____

_____

3. Which type of data analysis uses words and analytical reasoning? _____

_____

_____

4. What are the four categories of descriptive statistics?_____

_____

_____

5. What methods might be used to analyze qualitative data?_____

_____

_____

CRITICAL THINKING AND APPLICATION EXERCISES

1. Two classes took the same exam. The first class had a mean of 50 and standard deviation of 10. The second class also had a mean of 50, but the standard deviation was 5. Which class had the more homogeneous scores?

2. Consider a researcher who used religion and marital status as variables in a study. Should parametric or nonparametric inferential statistical tests be used to test the hypothesis? Why?

3. If a qualitative research study used grounded theory methodology, which method of data analysis would be most appropriate? Why?

4. Read a quantitative research report. Use the checklist on page 213 to critique the data analysis.

5. Read a qualitative research article. Use the checklist on page 217 to critique the data analysis.

23

Interpretation, Communication, and Use of Research Findings

LEARNING OBJECTIVES

After studying this chapter, you should be able to:

♦ Differentiate between statistical and clinical significance.

♦ Compare and contrast narrative and pictorial presentations of findings.

♦ Describe the relationship between findings and implications for nursing.

♦ Discuss oral, poster, and written formats used to communicate research findings.

♦ Identify barriers to using research.

♦ Discuss strategies for increasing the use of research.

♦ State the criteria for critiquing the research report.

CHAPTER OVERVIEW

This chapter presents the interpretation, communication, and utilization of research findings. It discusses the significance of findings as well as the difference between statistical and clinical significance. Presentation of the findings, forming conclusions, and deducing nursing implications are outlined. Formats for communicating research findings are described, and using research is discussed. Selected research utilization activities are presented, and pertinent questions to consider when critiquing a research report are listed.

♦ I. Introduction

A. The INTERPRETATION and communication of findings are the final steps in the research process

B. The researcher relies on creativity, logical reasoning, intelligence, and communication skills to arrive at conclusions and issue a report of the findings

C. The report may be presented orally at a conference or in writing as a research article

♦ II. Interpreting research findings

A. General information

1. Interpretation is the process by which the researcher examines, organizes, and attaches significance to the results obtained from data analysis; meaning is attached to the numbers in quantitative analysis and to the words in qualitative analysis

2. The researcher typically relies on introspection, logic, and intuition

3. The researcher should base the interpretation of findings on the purpose statement, conceptual or theoretical framework, hypotheses or research questions, literature review, population studied, and limitations of the research design

B. Significance of the findings

1. The researcher's interpretation of the data after analysis should yield one of three possible results

   a. Statistically significant findings that match the hypothesized findings are typically the easiest to interpret because the researcher will have already examined the variables and predicted the results

   b. Significant findings that contradict the hypothesized findings may result from the researcher's faulty logic or from flaws within the theory itself

   c. Nonsignificant findings may result from inappropriate methodology, a biased or small sample, threats to internal validity, unreliable or invalid instruments, weak statistical measures, faulty analysis, or theoretical weaknesses

2. The researcher must be especially careful to distinguish STATISTICAL SIGNIFICANCE from CLINICAL SIGNIFICANCE

   a. *Statistical significance* means that the null hypothesis has been rejected and any differences between groups are probably not the result of chance; statistical significance depends on sample size: the larger the sample, the greater the possibility of statistical significance

b. *Clinical significance* means that the findings may be useful in a clinical setting

C. Presentation of the findings

1. Findings usually are presented narratively and pictorially

a. A narrative presentation, which typically constitutes the text portion of a written report, should include specific information on the statistical test used, the results, and the probability value

b. A pictorial presentation typically includes illustrated graphs, HISTOGRAMS, pie charts, FREQUENCY POLYGONS, and tables

2. Tables used to summarize findings should be clearly labeled with titles that accurately identify the variables being presented; numbers should be consistently rounded to the same number of decimal places, with all decimal points aligned

3. When coordinating the narrative and illustrated portions of a report, the researcher should ensure that nothing in the text repeats what is in the illustrated portions and, conversely, that nothing in the illustrated portions repeats what is in the text

D. Forming conclusions

1. The researcher deduces conclusions from the current study findings coupled with information learned in previous research studies and the theoretical framework

2. When forming conclusions, the researcher must remember that research never proves anything—it merely lends support to a position

3. The researcher must always guard against allowing subjective judgments and biases to creep into conclusions

4. The researcher should also avoid extending conclusions beyond the available data

E. Nursing implications

1. When formulating conclusions, the researcher must provide practical suggestions for implementing the findings in nursing and for recommending future research

2. The researcher must consider which areas of nursing may be affected by the study findings and include at least one nursing implication for each conclusion drawn

3. Such implications typically focus on changes that should or should not be made in nursing practice, education, and research

♦ **III. Communicating research findings**

A. General information

1. The researcher must communicate findings to practitioners and researchers so that the study has an impact on nursing practice

2. To communicate the findings, the researcher must develop a RESEARCH REPORT that clearly and concisely describes the research problem, methodology, findings, and interpretation of the findings

CHECKLIST
Research report

Use the following questions as a guide to critiquing the research report of a study.

	Yes	No
• Considering the constraints on time and space, does the report include sufficient detail to permit a thorough critique of the study?	☐	☐
• Does the report include information on the research problem, framework, methodology, findings, and interpretation of the findings?	☐	☐
• Are tables and figures used to present the findings clearly titled and do they supplement the text?	☐	☐
• Is the report clear and concise?	☐	☐
• Is the report well organized and logically presented?	☐	☐
• Are implications for nursing practice, education, or research included in the conclusions?	☐	☐
• Does the researcher generalize about the results within the study's scope?	☐	☐

3. The report may be written or presented orally or pictorially in poster form; usually, an oral report presented at a conference is the quickest means of communicating the findings (see *Research report*)

B. Oral reports
  1. Presenting an oral report at a conference enables the researcher to disseminate the information quickly and to interact directly with the conference participants; however, because the number of conference attendees is typically limited, the researcher's ability to share the findings with a wide audience is limited
  2. Most oral presentations are limited to approximately 20 minutes; therefore, the researcher typically needs to give a condensed report of the findings and eliminate many of the study's details
  3. The researcher may rely on slides or transparencies to enhance the presentation and use an informal, lively tone when speaking

C. Poster presentations
  1. Poster presentations have become an increasingly popular way to communicate findings
  2. The researcher should remain with the poster to talk with the viewers and answer questions

3. The poster's appearance plays an important role in communicating the findings; it should incorporate color, diagrams, and graphs and should neatly and clearly present the content of the study in large, easy-to-read type

D. Written reports

1. The researcher may choose to communicate the research findings through a written report

2. Submitting a report for publication in a journal enables the researcher to communicate more detailed information about the study to a wider audience; however, depending on when and if the manuscript is accepted for publication, months or years may elapse before the report is finally published and read

3. When writing a report, the researcher must keep in mind the intended audience and use of the report

   a. For example, a report intended for publication in a nursing journal should contain appropriate language and should be concisely written to the desired article length

   b. As another example, a report intended for submission as a thesis or dissertation should demonstrate an in-depth understanding of the subject and the research process

4. A well-written report, which typically traces the study from beginning to end, has several parts

   a. An introductory discussion of the research problem and rationale for conducting the study

   b. A review of the literature used to develop the study and the framework that guided the study

   c. A detailed explanation of the methodology used to conduct the study, including information on the specific research design, sampling technique, and data collection method

   d. A presentation of the results, including the data analysis used and the researcher's interpretation of the findings

   e. The researcher's conclusions about the research findings and their implications for nursing

♦ IV. Using research findings

A. General information

1. The ultimate value of nursing research is the extent to which it is used in practice

2. The purpose of research utilization is to have the solutions identified through research used for the good of society

B. Barriers to research utilization

1. The majority of practicing nurses have not received instruction in research and lack the skills to evaluate and critique research reports

SEARCHING THE WEB
Nursing research and utilization

A newsletter, *Nursing Research and Research Utilization,* can be accessed at
http://usafsg.satx.disa.mil/~sgn/research/newltc09.htm#bkTOC.

2. Several years may pass between the time a researcher designs a study and practicing nurses learn about the results
3. Research reports may be seen as difficult to read and understand
4. Individuals and organizations are usually reluctant to change
5. Practicing nurses have not been rewarded for research utilization
6. Resources may not be available for conducting research or implementing findings
7. Researchers and practitioners fail to communicate and collaborate

C. Research utilization efforts
1. The Western Interstate Commission for Higher Education regional nursing research development project, initiated in the mid-1970s, was the first major effort focusing on nursing research utilization; nurses were given the opportunity to evaluate research aimed at solving practice problems
2. The Conduct and Utilization of Research in Nursing project, conducted from 1975 to 1980, sought to increase use of research findings by disseminating quality findings and facilitating their implementation
3. The Nursing Child Assessment Satellite Training project, begun in 1976, was educational and aimed at the practicing nurse; it supported the use of satellite communication for research dissemination
4. The Agency for Health Care Policy and Research of the U.S. Department of Health and Human Services' Public Health Service, in the early 1990s, developed clinical practice guidelines based on research

D. Strategies for increasing research use
1. Researchers should take the responsibility to conduct quality research in which the findings include clear implications for practice and are communicated clearly at every opportunity; researchers should also replicate studies and collaborate with practitioners
2. Educators should integrate research findings throughout the curriculum, stimulate intellectual curiosity and inquiry, and be actively involved in research activities
3. Administrators should offer emotional and financial support for efforts to use research and should reward its use
4. Practicing nurses should critically read research literature, attend professional meetings, collaborate with nursing researchers, and par-

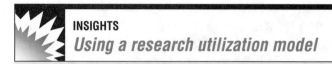

INSIGHTS

Using a research utilization model

In 1994, C. Stetler developed a research utilization model that can be used by an individual nurse. The model has six phases: preparation, validation, comparative evaluation, decision making, translation/application, and evaluation. This model is unique in that the perspective for research utilization is individual rather than organizational.

ticipate in research utilization projects (see *Using a research utilization model*)

POINTS TO REMEMBER

♦ Interpretation of research findings requires the use of introspection, logical reasoning, and intuition.

♦ Statistically significant findings suggest that differences between groups probably did not result from chance.

♦ Clinically significant findings are useful in the practice setting.

♦ All conclusions drawn from the findings should address the implications for nursing in relation to practice, education, and research.

♦ Findings must be communicated to and utilized by practitioners for research to have an effect on nursing practice.

♦ Research findings are typically communicated through a research report that may be written or presented orally or in poster form.

♦ Narrative presentations are typically supplemented by illustrated tables and graphs.

♦ Presenting a research report at a conference disseminates the findings rapidly; publishing a written report reaches a wider audience.

♦ The ultimate value of research is the extent to which it is used in practice.

STUDY QUESTIONS

To evaluate your understanding of this chapter, answer the following questions in the space provided; compare your responses with the correct answers in appendix B, pages 237 to 244.

1. What skills does the researcher use to interpret the findings?_____

_____

_____

2. What is the difference between statistical significance and clinical significance?_____

_____

_____

3. Why are nursing implications important? _____

_____

_____

4. What are three ways in which research findings might be communicated

_____

_____

5. How might the practicing nurse increase research utilization?_____

_____

_____

CRITICAL THINKING AND APPLICATION EXERCISES

1. In a research report, the findings were significant at the 0.01 level. The researcher concluded that the study proved that the hypothesis was correct. Was this a valid conclusion? Why?

2. In a research report, the author stated that the demographics of the sample were given in Table 1 and did not include the information in the narrative. Was this appropriate? Why?

3. View a poster presenting findings from a research study. What criteria might be used to evaluate the presentation? Why?

4. Read a quantitative research article. Use the checklist on page 223 to critique the report.

5. Read a qualitative research article. Use the checklist on page 223 to critique the report.

Glossary

Absolute zero point—point in measurement indicating a total absence of the item or attribute being measured; in interval level measurement, the zero point is arbitrary, not absolute

Abstract—brief summary of a research study

Accountability—assuming personal responsibility for actions and policies and accepting the consequences of one's behavior

Arbitration—process for settling labor disputes by involving a neutral third party, typically a labor relations expert

Associate nurse—nurse assigned to care for a primary nurse's patient when the primary nurse is unavailable, following the primary nurse's plan of care

Autocratic leadership—leadership style in which control rests entirely with the leader

Budget—funds allocated to an organization for ongoing and future use; an itemized summary of probable expenses and income for a given period; a tool for planning, monitoring and controlling costs and meeting expenses; a plan for use and evaluation of resources

Budget forecast—prediction of the activities of an organization over a set period of time, including such key items as expenses, revenues, materials, equipment, and personnel

Bureaucracy—complex organizational structure that relies on centralized power and authority; specialization of tasks; rigid rules, regulations, and hierarchy of authority; routine; formal communications; and detailed record keeping

Burnout—condition characterized by a lack of concern for one's work or profession that results from chronic, unrelieved, work-related stress

Capitol rate—hospital reimbursement system in which the hospital receives a flat rate for each member enrolled either through a health maintenance organization or a preferred provider organization

Case manager—registered nurse or other health care professional who has responsibility for coordinating care, from admission to discharge, for a specific group of patients

Case rate—hospital reimbursement system in which the hospital is paid a flat rate for each diagnosis

Centralized structure—organizational structure in which decisions are made at the top and handed down through management levels

Clinical significance—usefulness of a study's findings in a clinical setting

Closed-ended question—one that limits the respondent to a fixed number of answer choices

Cluster—large grouping of elements within a population

Collective bargaining—process of negotiation between employees (usually through a union or employee association) and organizational management in an attempt to agree on employment terms and conditions

Concept—idea to which a label or meaning is attached

Conceptual framework—abstract organization of concepts that provides direction for a research study

Confidentiality—protection of personal information against unnecessary or unauthorized disclosure

Continuous Quality Improvement (CQI)—outgrowth of Total Quality Management emphasizing a multidisciplinary team approach to planning or problem solving or both, carried out institutionally on a continuing basis

Cyclical work schedule—method of scheduling staff members using the same work schedule repeatedly

Database—large collection of information in a computer that can be rapidly retrieved, rearranged, and updated

Decentralized structure—employee-centered organizational structure in which decisions are made at the unit level

Decision package—device used in zero-based budgeting that lists all the activities of a given area, alternative ways of carrying out these activities and the cost for each, and the advantages of continuing and the consequences of discontinuing the activity; the activities are ranked from those essential to maintaining minimal operations to those nonessential but desirable

Decision rules—criteria used in Vroom and Yetton model of decision making to identify an appropriate management style in a specific situation

Decision tree—diagram of the problem-solving process that identifies the primary problem and at least two alternative problems

Deductive reasoning—process by which specifics are inferred from general principles; relies on the accuracy of the general principles to arrive at valid conclusions

Democratic leadership—leadership style in which control is shared equally by the leader and the group members

Descriptive research—study in which the researcher accurately portrays the characteristics of a particular individual, situation, or group to outline existence, determine the frequency with which something occurs, or classify information

Diagnosis-related group (DRG)—system that classifies the patient by age, medical diagnosis, and surgical procedure, to predict the use of hospital resources and length of stay and to set predetermined Medicare reimbursement rates

Dissertation—original research study written by a candidate for a doctoral degree

Driving forces—forces that move the target of change in the desired direction

Effect size—statistical expression describing the magnitude of a relationship between two variables

Element—basic unit that makes up the sample and the population about which information is collected

Empirical evidence—data based on objective observation or experience

Empirical testing—objective analysis, typically using statistical techniques, of evidence gained objectively through the senses

Empirical-rational strategy—strategy for handling minimal resistance to change; can be used to persuade the target to accept a rational change

based on information about the change that is in the target's self-interest

Expenditures—monies listed on a budget as spent; also known as expenses

Exploratory research—preliminary study conducted to gain insight, discover ideas, or increase knowledge in a particular area

Feedback—in systems theory, the analysis and interpretation of output with the purpose of either reactivating or changing the system

Frequency polygon—graphic representation of a frequency distribution that uses dots connected by straight lines to depict the frequency (number) of data identified on a horizontal axis

Gain sharing—method of allowing employees to share in the economic success of a for-profit health care institution; stock ownership and profit sharing are similar options

"Great man" theory—leadership theory holding that the great leaders are born and that the qualities of effective leadership are inherited and cannot be taught or learned

Grievance—substantial employee complaint to management, usually involving working condition or contract violations

study or the person who developed the theory

Self-governance—control of nursing services and their costs by nurses

Shared governance—means of involving staff nurses in all nursing-related decisions through participation in a formal nursing staff organization that establishes standards of practice, quality, education, management, research, and professionalism; the organizational structure consists of a nurse executive board and various councils and their committees

Situational theory—leadership theory proposing that essential traits for a leader vary depending on particular situations

Span of control—number of employees a manager can effectively oversee

Staff position—advisory or service person with little or no decision-making authority, depicted in the organizational chart by dotted or horizontal lines

Staffing—function and process of determining and securing the nursing personnel required to provide safe, quality patient care over a 24-hour period

Standard—level of optimal performance that defines the scope and degree of nursing care necessary to ensure quality of nursing care

Statistical significance—usefulness of a study's findings based on rejection of the null hypothesis and on the probability that differences between groups do not result from chance

Team leader—nurse assigned to care for a group of patients with the help of other nurses (team nurses) and ancillary personnel; he or she is responsible for supervising and coordinating all care provided by the team members

Theoretical definition—general, abstract meaning that the researcher ascribes to a variable

Theory—formal set of interrelated concepts and propositions used to describe, explain, predict, control, or understand an aspect of reality

Thesis—formal research study written by a candidate for a master's degree

Throughput—in systems theory, the processing or transformation of input

Total Quality Management (TQM)—system of management that focuses on those processes that ensure organization efficiency, effectiveness, and quality through organizational teamwork and excellence

Trait theory—leadership theory positing that qualities of effective leadership can be identified, taught, and learned

Transformational theory—leadership theory proposing that leaders and followers interact to achieve higher levels of motivation

True score—most accurate value obtainable if the instrument were perfect

Unfreezing—first step in the three-step process of planned change that results from the imbalance in the driving and restraining forces; the status quo is disrupted and new patterns of behavior must be developed

Utilization Review Accreditation Committee (URAC)—committee that evaluates a hospital's resource allocation by examining such factors as patient admissions (to the hospital and to a particular unit within the hospital), length of stay, and problems after discharge, including readmissions

Variable—characteristic of a person or object that differs among members of the population

Variable work schedule—method of scheduling staff members by providing each nurse unit with a minimum number of staff members and increasing or decreasing that number according to the workload

Vulnerable subject—any individual whose rights are at high risk of violation during a research study; vulnerable populations include children and those who are mentally impaired, terminally ill, or institutionalized

Zero-based budgeting—budget preparation in which all expenses of a department, organization, or division must be rejustified annually to be reincluded in the next year's budget

Answers to Study Questions

CHAPTER 1

1. Values clarification is the Z-step process of examining personal beliefs, values, and principles and the degree to which one acts in accordance with them on a regular basis.
2. An organization's structure is determined by its operative organizational theory.
3. Classical organizational theory holds that the role of management is to increase production by closely supervising the work of others.
4. A parental leader fosters obedience and dependency in group members.
5. Planning is the most critical management function.

CHAPTER 2

1. Key elements of a bureaucracy include a centralized authority structure, highly specialized division of labor, rigid hierarchy of management, rigid rules and regulations, routine, formal communications, and detailed record keeping.
2. The Hawthorne experiment refers to research that discovered that various psychological and social factors in the work situation exerted more influence on productivity than did actual physical conditions.
3. The hallmark of modern organizational theory is the systems framework.
4. Modern organizational theory focuses on organizational processes rather than on structure.

CHAPTER 3

1. The philosophy of an organization forms the basis of the formal organizational structure.
2. Organizational structure can be centralized or decentralized.
3. Organizational climate refers to the employees' perception of the workplace.
4. Official, voluntary, and proprietary health care organizations are types of organizations categorized by their major source of funding.

CHAPTER 4

1. Case nursing is considered the oldest approach to patient care.
2. Functional nursing reflects a bureaucratic, centralized organization.
3. A team leader is responsible for managing the care of a group of patients. He or she assigns personnel, plans and evaluates the nursing care provided by the

team, and reports to the nurse-manager.

4. Primary nursing reflects a decentralized organizational structure.

5. A critical path refers to a time frame used in managed care and takes into account the usual length of stay, interventions and their timing, resources needed, and expected patient outcomes.

CHAPTER 5

1. According to the "great man" theory, leadership is inherited and cannot be taught or learned; that is, people are born to lead.

2. According to the trait theory, leadership qualities can be identified and taught to others. Specific personality traits are essential to leadership, including intelligence, knowledge, skill, energy and enthusiasm, initiative, self-confidence, patience, persistence, and empathy.

3. Group performance depends on the leader choosing an appropriate leadership style based on the four basic elements (organization, climate, leader characteristics, and follower characteristics) of the situation.

4. The tridimensional leadership effectiveness model focuses on leader behavior, group maturity, and leader effectiveness.

5. Transformational leadership attempts to create a meaningful, inspirational, and motivational workplace.

CHAPTER 6

1. Planned change incorporates predetermination of goals, participative management, a change agent, and a target for change.

2. Win-lose is a situation in which one side dominates the other through superior power. Lose-lose involves resolution through avoidance, withdrawal, compromise, or bribery with an outcome unsatisfactory to both sides. Win-win is an outcome satisfactory to both sides.

3. Kinesics is the use of body motions; proxemics, the use of space; paralinguistics, the use of verbal expressions, such as "ah" and "um," touch, and physical or environmental factors or both.

4. Legitimate power derives from a formal position of authority; referent power is based on association with a powerful leader; expert power resides in the use of knowledge, skill, and expertise; reward power is the ability to confer privilege or favor; coercive power is the ability to compel others to comply by withholding rewards or applying sanctions.

5. Optimizing strategy involves examining all solutions and choosing the best one possible; satisficing strategy involves selecting a solution that, although not ideal, meets the minimal standards for resolution.

CHAPTER 7

1. Team management, described as a great concern for both production and people, is considered ideal because it emphasizes the involvement of employees in all aspects of the managerial process.
2. The focus of management is enhanced productivity, which is achieved through uniform standards, effective feedback, and rewards for performance. Involving employees in those processes that affect them can increase employee commitment to enhanced productivity.
3. Fiedler's contingency model of managerial effectiveness is the only model to explore the concept of power as a key variable.
4. Participative management is possible only in a decentralized organizational structure.
5. Organizational teamwork and individual empowerment are essential to a Total Quality Management approach. However, neither are possible without managerial and administrative commitment to individual employee autonomy in decision making.

CHAPTER 8

1. Assertiveness helps increase self-awareness, self-confidence, and maturity, which are essential in establishing clear priorities and expectations, and in delegating, through effective communication, the authority to carry out a delegated task. Priority setting

and delegation are key to effective time management, risk management, and performance appraisal.
2. Bench marking is the practice of measuring the overall effectiveness of a process by comparing it to similar processes. In performance appraisal, bench marking involves selection of the best example of performance as a criterion to measure related performances. In Continuous Quality Improvement, bench marking involves selection of a standard of excellence in a process or a procedure and using that standard to measure related processes or procedures.
3. The two standards emphasized by both Quality Assurance and Continuous Quality Improvement programs are outcome and process standards.
4. A mentor provides an individual with direction, counseling, and ongoing support in career development. Having a mentor paves the way for developing self-confidence and commitment to personal and professional self-actualization, which is the highest form of motivation.

CHAPTER 9

1. The desired outcome of any organizational budget is the optimal use of resources.
2. In zero-based budgeting, expenditures for the previous year are irrelevant; each year the budget starts at zero. Incremental budgeting uses previous year expen-

ditures as the basis for the current budget.

3. In any organization, the two principal expenditures in an operating budget are personnel and supplies and equipment.

CHAPTER 10

1. Staffing is determined by the number and mix of personnel available, patient census, type of patient care delivery system in use, and levels of patient acuity.

2. Patient classification systems, if properly managed, enable nurse managers to objectively quantify nursing care in terms of the "costing out" of nursing services. Costing out nursing services is essential for justifying the need for skilled nursing care and obtaining reimbursement for that care.

3. Decentralized staffing relates to Continuous Quality Improvement in that accountability is developed from the point of service upward through the administrative levels. Accountability for staffing, for example, takes place at the nursing unit level.

CHAPTER 11

1. Economic changes have resulted in federally mandated efforts to reduce expenditures; increased consumer demand for quality service; increased competition among health care organizations; and demand for cost containment, cost-effectiveness, and

health care provider excellence and accountability.

2. Demographic changes are necessitating a shift in nursing practice from hospital-based to community-based care, creating more independent and diversified nursing roles that require strong leadership and management skills.

3. The American Nurses Association's (ANA) call for health care reform includes a restructuring to enhance patient access, a minimum standard health care package for all, decreased costs through appropriate use of managed care, case management, and ongoing evaluation.

CHAPTER 12

1. The National Labor Relations Board resolves disputes between an employer and a bargaining unit.

2. Health care organizations, because of their responsibility for patient safety, must be given 10 days' notice before a strike can take place.

3. Providing employees with a financial incentive by allowing them to share in the profits of an institution is one way of making employees more conscious of efficiency measures and measures to reduce waste.

4. Inadequate staffing can cause discontent, frustration, stress, poor morale, increased turnover, and absenteeism.

CHAPTER 13

1. The primary goal of nursing research is to develop a specialized, scientifically based body of knowledge.
2. Basic research is done to advance the body of knowledge, whereas applied research is done to remedy a particular problem.
3. Florence Nightingale furthered nursing research by emphasizing the importance of systematic observation, data collection, environmental factors, and statistical analyses.
4. A researcher might conduct a pilot study to minimize the possibility of having significant difficulties with the major study.
5. All nurses need to critique previously conducted and newly proposed research.

CHAPTER 14

1. Experimental studies noted for unethical treatment of human subjects include Nazi medical experiments, the Tuskegee syphilis study, the Jewish Chronic Disease Hospital study, and the Willowbrook hepatitis study.
2. The Nuremburg Code resulted from the unethical experimentation spotlighted during the Nazi criminal trials.
3. The three ethical principles relevant to research are respect, beneficence, and justice.
4. Human rights requiring protection are self-determination, privacy, anonymity or confidentiality, fair treatment, and protection from harm.

CHAPTER 15

1. Identification of the research problem is important because it provides direction for the entire study.
2. Nursing practice, literature, theory, and interactions with peers and researchers might be sources for research problems.
3. Factors to be considered when selecting a research problem are its significance, researchability, feasibility, and interest to the researcher.
4. A purpose statement may be interrogative or declarative.

CHAPTER 16

1. A literature review is done to lay the foundation for the research or to compare and contrast the literature with the findings from the current study.
2. A review may help the researcher to identify or refine the problem, strengthen the rationale for the research, develop a framework, provide a useful approach to conducting the study, and explain or support the findings.
3. The researcher reviews research findings, theoretical information, methodological information, opinion articles, and anecdotal descriptions.
4. Indexes are the researcher's main source for manually locating articles published in journals.

5. A computer search is more current and less time-consuming than a manual search; it also allows concepts to be combined in the search.

CHAPTER 17

1. Nursing researchers are particularly interested in the key concepts of person, environment, health, and nursing.
2. A schematic model uses boxes and arrows; a mathematical model uses letters, numbers, and mathematical symbols.
3. Conceptual frameworks are based on specific concepts and propositions; theoretical frameworks are based on a theory.
4. Nursing theories used to guide nursing research include Roy's "Adaptation Model," Orem's "Self-Care Model," Rogers's "Science of Unitary Human Beings," and Neuman's "Health-Care Systems Model."
5. Theories borrowed from other disciplines used to guide nursing research include Bandura's "Social Learning Theory," Lazarus's and Selye's stress theories, Spielberger's anxiety theory, and Melzack's and Wall's pain theory.
6. Common problems related to conceptual and theoretical frameworks include use of an inappropriate or unidentified framework, use of a framework that is disconnected from the study, and use of multiple frameworks within the same study.

CHAPTER 18

1. A variable is a concept examined in a research study; a hypothesis predicts the relationship between the variables.
2. The theoretical definition of a variable is broad and abstract and is derived from literature; the operational definition reflects the procedures that the researcher performs in experimental research.
3. The independent variable is the presumed cause or influencing factor and is manipulated by the researcher to examine the effect on the dependent variable.
4. A researcher would use a complex hypothesis to predict a relationship among two or more independent variables and two or more dependent variables.
5. Research questions guiding qualitative studies are usually broader and more abstract than those in quantitative research.

CHAPTER 19

1. Quantitative research is based on reductionism and uses variables that are analyzed as numbers; qualitative research is based on holism and uses concepts that are analyzed as words.
2. Threats to internal validity include history, maturation, testing, instrumentation, mortality or attrition, and selection bias.
3. The characteristics of a true experimental design are manipulation, control, and randomization.